Medicine over Mind

Critical Issues in Health and Medicine

Edited by Rima D. Apple, University of Wisconsin–Madison, and Janet Golden, Rutgers University, Camden

Growing criticism of the U.S. healthcare system is coming from consumers, politicians, the media, activists, and healthcare professionals. Critical Issues in Health and Medicine is a collection of books that explores these contemporary dilemmas from a variety of perspectives, among them political, legal, historical, sociological, and comparative, and with attention to crucial dimensions such as race, gender, ethnicity, sexuality, and culture.

For a list of titles in the series, see the last page of the book.

Medicine over Mind

Mental Health Practice in the Biomedical Era

Dena T. Smith

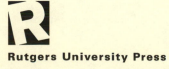

Rutgers University Press

New Brunswick, Camden, and Newark, New Jersey, and London

Library of Congress Cataloging-in-Publication Data
Names: Smith, Dena T., author.
Title: Medicine over mind : mental health practice in the biomedical era /
    Dena T. Smith.
Other titles: Critical issues in health and medicine.
Description: New Brunswick : Rutgers University Press, 2019. | Series:
    Critical issues in health and medicine | Includes bibliographical references.
Identifiers: LCCN 2019002220 | ISBN 9780813598666
Subjects: | MESH: Psychiatry—trends | Psychoanalytic Therapy—methods |
    Psychotropic Drugs | Mental Disorders—therapy
Classification: LCC RC454 | NLM WM 100 | DDC 616.89—dc23
LC record available at https://lccn.loc.gov/2019002220

A British Cataloging-in-Publication record for this book is available from the British Library.

♾ The paper used in this publication meets the requirements of the American National
Standard for Information Sciences—Permanence of Paper for Printed Library Materials,
ANSI Z39.48-1992.

www.rutgersuniversitypress.org

Manufactured in the United States of America

About twenty-five years ago, I held a small gathering in our Brooklyn apartment for my mother to celebrate her successful dissertation defense. It was modest. I was thirteen. At the end of the afternoon, one of the women in her writing group turned to me and my younger brother and asked whether we'd ever become doctors like our mom. Offering an emphatic "no," I gently rolled my eyes at such an unreasonable query. My little brother, one of the smartest people I know, offered a "maybe" and became a comedian; life is filled with uncertainties. This book is for my mom because what I know for sure is that without her, for so many reasons, this project would not have been possible.

Contents

Medicine over Mind

Under the Influence
of the Biomedical Model

On a hot July day, I arrived at a modern Midtown Manhattan office building to interview Dr. King. A bit early for our midday meeting, I sifted through an impressive collection of *New Yorker* magazines, cooled off, and gathered my thoughts to the familiar humming of a white-noise machine. Having spent significant time in psychiatrists' and psychologists' waiting rooms all over New York City, I'd developed a game of trying to predict what awaited me behind office doors. I knew little about Dr. King's practice except that she was a psychiatrist and a psychoanalyst, which meant she was trained in psychopharmacology and diagnosis (tools of the mainstream psychiatric trade today) as well as in the psychodynamic tradition of in-depth talk therapy (a rarity for a psychiatrist today). So I expected she would have an analytic couch on which patients are meant to recline as they unburden themselves of conflict-laden thoughts and desires. Her office would also probably be marked with icons of biomedical psychiatry like a copy (often more than one edition) of the *Diagnostic and Statistical Manual of Mental Disorders* (DSM), the guidebook for classifying disorders according to symptom sets that has become the symbol of biomedical psychiatry. Perhaps Dr. King would have a prescription pad on a desk or side table—or maybe the more understated type, she would tuck it away in a desk drawer.

Dr. King emerged promptly from her office and greeted me unceremoniously, and within a few minutes we were engaged in a somewhat awkward interchange. I endeavored to provide some background on the project, which had been a generally mundane process with interviewees—most practitioners paid little attention to my fairly rehearsed narrative while I surveyed their office landscapes to see how accurate my waiting-room predictions had been. The first few minutes of my meetings with practitioners often involved their jokes about difficulties with institutional review boards approving research or play-ful inquiries as to whether they were "signing their life away" by agreeing to participate in my study. A handful asked probing questions about my interest in psychiatric paradigms and practice, but most followed along once I began to explain why I was interviewing mental health practitioners. Dr. King, however, interrupted me to inquire, "This is for psychology?" Wondering if she hadn't read the project description in my introductory email, I replied, "sociology," as I tucked her signed consent forms under other papers on my clipboard and attempted a return to my explanation of the study. But she interjected again: "So, you're still doing sociology?" "Yes, mhm," I replied, feeling slightly off-kilter now and wondering what prompted this aside. Trying once more to move beyond our introduction, a short pause gave her an opening to add, "You should go to medical school and become a psychiatrist." Being on the spot about my field and my perspective was not an entirely unfamiliar feeling in encounters with mental health practitioners, who, I learned early on, tended to try to turn the tables at the outset by asking me questions, a role they no doubt felt more comfortable playing. I chuckled a bit self-consciously at Dr. King's suggestion, alluded to the fact that I'd once considered becoming a clinician, and veered us back on track by asking her why she decided to become a psychiatrist, my typical opening inquiry. She permitted our conversation to advance, but the interchange lingered in my mind, and I left feeling uncertain about its mean-ing, particularly since Dr. King was insightful and helpful for the remainder of our meeting.

That evening I inspected my field notes as I began transcribing my conver-sation with Dr. King. In the margins I had scrawled a less than entirely legible note to myself that Dr. King referenced *Love and Its Place in Nature*, Jonathan Lear's (1990) book of reflections on psychoanalysis, which I had not read. Prac-titioners would regularly allude to various texts, both of their own and of others' authorship (and sometimes suggest I read them), as a way to explain their orientations to the field, or an allegiance to a particular style of treatment, to educate me on something I clearly wasn't exposed to, and sometimes because they'd gleaned my areas of interest. I transcribed my conversation with Dr. King through a lasting sense of confusion and even irritation at her blunt suggestion, without any understanding of me as a person, that I switch careers.

A month or so later, still sensing I was missing something since that open-ing exchange with Dr. King felt out of context for our overall relatively amica-ble conversation, I had the occasion to peruse *Love and Its Place in Nature: A*

Philosophical Interpretation of Freudian Psychoanalysis. I returned to the recording of my conversation with Dr. King. About fifteen minutes in, I asked her whether she thinks the kind of pain and suffering her patients bring into treatment can ever be useful. I asked this question of all my interviewees as it often elicited a discussion of a range of issues around treatment and etiology. That's when Dr. King referenced Lear's discussion of attitudes toward psychotropic medication, the moment I'd noted in my field notes:

> At one point he says, you know, do we really wanna take away that depression, that pain? You know, because that's an opening for the self-exploration. And I remember reading that and thinking like how off base that was and that if somebody is in pain and we have a treatment for that, like a medicine, that we should help them. And so, is pain useful? Yeah, pain is sometimes useful in that it, you know, it can force people to look at things, but I think we have to be very, what's the word? *Respectful* of that. Because we also want people to not be in pain. And I think that when people realize that we're helping them with their pain, our alliance gets better and we can probably do better analysis.

In an almost indignant tone, Dr. King described the idea of using pain as an opening for self-exploration as "off base." One of the philosophical and treatment goals of psychoanalysis is to explore suffering, often conceptualized as internal conflict, and to uncover its derivations. Such a practice indeed goes against much of what the biomedical model teaches—when there's an intervention, use it, when medication is helpful, prescribe it. When Dr. King says, "When people realize we're helping them with their pain," she's referencing the use of psychotropic medications to assuage symptoms as swiftly as possible.

As I revisited this moment in our conversation several times, it became clear that Dr. King's outrage at Lear's statement about the utility of symptoms was more than a philosophical disagreement about the role of pain and suffering in treatment—it was a comment at the heart of her thinking. To her, Lear's comment was "off base" because it's not the responsible approach of a medical doctor to allow a patient to suffer when there's a medical intervention, though she agrees that pain can "force people to look at things." Lear's approach was also out of sync with Dr. King's ideas about etiology. She was clear that both "nature and nurture" are responsible for the kinds of conditions her patients experience, but "people are born with genes," she told me, and "all psychiatric mental issues are somehow dictated by neural substrate." She added, "And then you go through life and you have attachment considerations that affect how you develop, and you have environmental accidents that happen to you in life like who you get for first grade or whether you're traumatized." Despite the importance of other factors, biological vulnerability is the foundation, and symptoms that extend from such susceptibility can presumably be treated with medication.

In reexamining my conversation with Dr. King, I was also reminded of what other practitioners (mostly those with dual training in psychiatry and psychoanalysis) like Dr. Park told me when we discussed her treatment approach: "Someone's interested in meaning and soul and mind, we're gonna get there and there's no particular advantage in having them writhing around with treatable pain." Like Dr. King, Dr. Park feels it's important to manage acute symptoms first, and to get to the murkier questions of meaning later. Dr. Nelson likewise explained her sense of responsibility to act in line with her medical training. "If someone fits into a DSM diagnosis that medicine treats," she explained, "I basically feel like it's my obligation as a physician to offer it up." The biomedical model is the primary way of dealing with symptoms, especially if a patient meets the criteria for a DSM diagnosis. Psychopharmacological intervention might prepare a patient for a more in-depth talk therapy. Yet, as Dr. Park's wording subtly alluded to, patients will eventually get to "meaning, and soul and mind"—but only *if* they're interested.

And yet these anecdotes are not a fair representation of the thinking of Drs. King, Nelson, or Park; as psychoanalysts, they are deeply interested in patients' experiences, which they made very clear at other points in our conversation. Despite her biomedical worldview, Dr. King describes psychoanalysis as having drawn her to psychiatry in the first place. She has a small practice, and sees none of her patients for medications only; in fact, a number are in a traditional, four-times-per-week psychoanalysis. And only about half of her patients take medication at all, which is much less than is typical of a psychiatry practice. But in her narrative as well as the majority of my interviewees' descriptions of their field and practice, it is evident that the biomedical model maintains its primacy over psychodynamic thinking.

Most of the practitioners I spoke with believe, some deeply, in the biomedical model and identify with its fundamental principles. As such, when individuals experience psychiatric troubles that interfere with their professional life or interpersonal relationships or when their general functioning is impaired, medication not only is an option but is generally described as a necessary intervention. Even the doctors I spoke with who practice largely outside the biomedical model—some are trained as psychologists rather than as medical doctors—practice in a field impacted by the forces of medicalization; their sessions take place in the context of managed care, in a field where pharmaceutical companies exert pressure to prescribe psychotropic medications, in a larger cultural context in which patients often prefer and even demand medicinal treatment for their troubles, and where training to practice in-depth talk therapy is a rarity.

It was in this context that Dr. King's suggestion that I become a psychiatrist was no longer puzzling. In fact, it made perfect sense. Her advice was not meant to be antagonistic; it just made good sense because she sees the biomedical model as the right way to think through the issues I described as central to this project. In fact, Dr. King was not the only psychiatrist I interviewed to suggest that I train in psychiatry, although she was the first and certainly the most candid. As Dr. King is a seasoned psychoanalyst, her critique of Lear initially struck me as paradoxical. But practitioners trained extensively in Freudian theory, who value the principles of psychodynamic psychotherapy, would often say of medication, "People can actually be more thoughtful, more reflective when they're not so miserable," or medication "can play a very, very beneficial role . . . it opens up the thinking and in the opening up of the thinking is typically better capacity to do a good psychotherapy." According to the majority of the practitioners in my study, using two of the most powerful tools of the mental health trade—talk therapy and medication—in combination is simply the best course of treatment. Yet the biomedical model often wins out over other forms of treatment, even though psychodynamic thinking and principles figure prominently in many practices where patients are also prescribed medications.

It wasn't just around medication that I encountered these seemingly contradictory statements, often over the course of a single interview. The most psychoanalytically oriented practitioners talked about the importance of the DSM, frequently in the same breath as they critiqued and sometimes denigrated it. Over approximately forty hours of interviews with forty-three practitioners, the majority of whom are psychoanalysts, I heard repeatedly about the prominence of the biomedical model in their practice. This book is the result of my efforts to understand how even practitioners trained in ways seemingly at odds with its assumptions have taken up or worked within the biomedical model. I explore how mental health practitioners trained in diverse schools navigate a biomedical world.

Mental Health Treatment in the Biomedical Model

This book follows in the long tradition in sociology, anthropology, and history of examining the forces that impact the mental health fields, the conceptualization of mental health and illness, and the consequences of both for patients and practitioners. In particular, I investigate how mental health practitioners experience and perpetuate the ongoing process of medicalization. They practice in a field wherein emotions, experiences, and psychological troubles are conceptualized as medical problems—specifically as disorders—and considered in need of medical intervention (Conrad 1992; Conrad and Schneider 1980; Freidson 1970; Horwitz 2002a; Scull 2015; Shorter 1998; Zola 1972). At the same time as psychiatry came under the purview of the medical model (and partly because of it), psychiatry's psychoanalytic roots withered for a range of reasons beginning in the 1970s, culminating in a complete reinvention of diagnostic standards and treatment approaches over the course of the 1980s (Horwitz 2002a). Some of the forces driving this dramatic shift, like discrete diagnosis and psycho-pharmacology, were endemic to the field, while others were largely the result of external forces like managed care, the increased influence of pharmaceutical companies, and demand from consumers for medicinal treatments (Conrad 2005; Hale 1995; Horwitz 2002a; Light and Levine 1988).

By the late 1980s psychiatry exemplified the biomedical thinking and treat-ment that permeated American medicine,[1] prompting scholars to describe the state of affairs with terms like "medicalization," "biomedicalization" (Clarke et al. 2003), and even "pharmaceuticalization" (Abraham 2010), which, partic-ularly in psychiatry, accurately represents the central role of psychopharma-cology. A lynchpin of the biomedical model in psychiatry was the third edition of the DSM, which the American Psychiatric Association released in 1980. A massive volume meant as the guidebook for psychiatrists in assessing their patients' symptoms and for research psychiatrists in ensuring the validity of the conditions they measure, its publication was an integral moment in the ascen-dance of the biomedical model in psychiatry—so central in fact that Horwitz (2002a) dubbed the post–DSM-III era "diagnostic psychiatry." Discrete diagnosis shifted the focus in psychiatry to disorders that matched the kinds of condi-tions doctors in other fields of medicine treated and allowed mental health prac-titioners to envision patients as suffering from disorders—the kind that could be treated with psychopharmacological interventions.

In psychiatry, psychotropic medications became the treatment of choice by the late 1980s when drugs like Prozac came to be seen as magic bullets for a range of conditions related to depression and anxiety. Between the 1980s and the turn of the twenty-first century, the reliance on pharmaceuticals expanded significantly (Busfield 2010; Williams, Martin, and Gabe 2011). The use of anti-depressant medications tripled between 1988 and 2000, and by the second decade of the twenty-first century nearly one in ten Americans had been pre-scribed an antidepressant drug. According to the Centers for Disease Control and Prevention's National Center for Health Statistics, 12.7 percent of Americans reported taking an antidepressant drug in the past thirty days, which represented a drastic increase from prior survey periods (Pratt, Brody, and Gu 2017). In the 2005–2008 survey period, it was 11 percent, in the 1999–2002 survey period, the percentage was 6.4 percent, and in the 1988–1994 period, only 1.8 percent. For more than a decade, antidepressants have been the third most prescribed class of medications in the United States (only behind antihyperlipidemic agents used for high cholesterol and analgesics for pain relief), and the most frequently used by those eighteen to forty-four years old (Pratt, Brody, and Gu 2011). And between the late 1980s and 2008, the rate of antidepressant use in the United States increased nearly 400 percent (Pratt, Brody, and Gu 2011). Even antipsychotic prescriptions, which were once reserved for a very small range of the most severe psychiatric illnesses, are on the rise for use not only in treating bipolar disorder but for a range of other diagnoses like depression and anxiety; Abilify, for example, is one of the top ten prescribed drugs in the United States. While it is not mental health professionals alone who prescribe these medications, as much of the psychotropic prescribing in the United States happens in the offices of internists and general practitioners, these trends indicate that the most common treatment for psychiatric symptoms today is medication.

As a field that was just a few decades ago ruled by psychodynamic principles and whose central intervention was ongoing, deep exploration of the psyche, the shift toward biological thinking and a diagnostic model radically altered the nature of psychiatric practice and had ripple effects into all mental health fields. The National Institute of Mental Health reported in 2008 that a significant percentage of Americans, 13.4 percent, had received care for a mental health problem (increased from 12.8 percent in 2004), but the kinds of treatments they received were less likely than ever before to involve talk therapy. Over the course of the 1990s and into the twenty-first century, talk therapy became an even less frequently used intervention. Anchored in what were lauded as cutting-edge pharmacological tools and a new classificatory system—and with the backing of pharmaceutical and insurance companies—psychiatry came to rely on somewhat ephemeral notions of neurochemical, biological etiology. The backdrop against which American psychiatry was practiced, even by the 1990s, looked radically different than it had just ten years earlier. Pharmaceutical companies and managed care only increased in power, and patient consumers, influenced by the pervasiveness of the biomedical model in American scientific and medical culture, also pushed for formal diagnoses and medicinal treatments (Conrad 2005, 2007). Furedi (2004, 101) summarizes the two key trends: "Since the 1980s, opposition to medicalisation has been minimal. This period has also seen an unprecedented level of the medicalisation of social experience." Some practitioners do push back against what they see as an encroachment by the biomedical model on their autonomy to practice as they see fit and against the dismissal of the basic principles of talk therapy; there is some resistance to medicalization particularly from practitioners trained in psychodynamic psychotherapy, but it is certainly diminished and much less active than ever before (Smith 2014).

Emblematic of the widespread acceptance of the biomedical model in psychiatry was the dramatic reduction in the hours residents spent learning the skills of talk therapy in favor of teaching diagnosis and psychopharmacology (Shorter 1997, 307), which had wide-ranging impacts on practice. By the late 1990s the percentage of psychiatrists providing some kind of psychotherapy to all patients was only 19.1 percent. Its use was reduced even further by the beginning of the twenty-first century; by 2005 only 10.8 percent provided psychotherapy (Kaplan 2008, 1). Today, even when nonmedicinal treatment is offered, it is likely to be cognitive behavioral therapy (CBT)[2] or one of a range of short-term, problem-focused talk therapies rather than more in-depth verbal therapies like psychodynamic psychotherapy or psychoanalysis (McWilliams 2000).[3]

Given these shifts over a relatively short period of time, late twentieth-century psychiatry was a field divided and replete with professional competition between, on the one hand, those who believed deeply in the efficacy of psychodynamic treatments and, on the other, those who saw the promise of psychopharmacology and evidence-based medicine more broadly (Horwitz 2002a; Klitzman 1995; Shorter 1998). Luhrmann (2001, 158) aptly captured the divide in hospitals when she described the psychoanalyst as the "wise wizard of insight" and the diagnostician as "fearless investigator of [scientific] truth." Yet nearly two decades into the twenty-first century, with the DSM-III and the mainstream use of antidepressants nearly forty years behind us, biomedical psychiatry is a fait accompli.

Despite the dominance of the biomedical model, we know little about what it's like for mental health practitioners in a biomedical world, where the voices and the power of psychoanalysts are largely absent from hospital settings. Medicalization requires maintenance; it is an ongoing process (Zola 1983, 295), and practitioners' beliefs and practices contribute to the continued success and authority of the biomedical model. Like Conrad (2007, 4), I'm interested in the "social underpinnings" and the "social implications" of the biomedical model; the experiences of mental health practitioners offer insight into both, as they treat a range of conditions from depression to bipolar disorder, as well as what many have called "problems in living" and "the worried well," yet their voices are relatively absent. We know little about how practitioners—both those who practice squarely within the biomedical model as well as those who practice talk therapy, particularly psychodynamic psychotherapy and psychoanalysis—experience their field today. How do they navigate practice within a well-established biomedical culture?

This Is a Book about Practitioners

This is a book about forty-three mental health practitioners' experiences in a biomedical world. It is not a book about mental health treatment or psychiatry at large, although my interviewees offer insight into the kinds of experiences, struggles, and attitudes others with similar training likely experience, and into some of the key issues in private-practice psychiatry and psychology. I echo Freidson's (1970, 19) largely unexplored call for investigations of practice in his groundbreaking work on the medical professions. "It is in the realities of practice," he argues, "rather than in the classroom that we find the empirical materials for clarifying and articulating the actual rather than the imputed or hoped-for nature of the professional role." How do the models doctors learn in training actually play out in their interactions with and their thinking about patients? Likewise, the physician Eric Cassell (2004, vii) argues, in his critique of modern medicine, "theories of medicine are exemplified by the actions of doctors." In the Bourdieuian sense, doctors' practice is engagement in cultural replication as they put their training into action. This is also true for psychoanalysts who seek to maintain a foothold for in-depth talking treatments in a largely biomedical field. How do psychiatrists and other mental health practitioners engage with their notions of etiology and appropriate treatment once they are in private practice, in offices away from the gaze of supervisors, once they settle in as seasoned professionals? How does their practice reproduce the lessons of their training well beyond their residency and internship years?

In practitioners' narratives are insights into what McGann, Hutson, and Rothman (2011) refer to as "medicalization-in-action." Though medicalization may be advanced in psychiatry, it relies on the continued support of practitioners, whom Conrad (2005, 5) dubbed the "gatekeepers" of medicalization as they remain largely in control of diagnosis and responsible for treatment decisions, even if both are under the influence of managed care, pharmaceutical companies, and pressures from patient-consumers. DSM diagnosis is a key feature of mental health practice in the age of evidence-based medicine, a tool of standardization. Timmermans and Berg point specifically to the importance of examining what standards like the DSM "*do* in medical practice" (2003a, 22, emphasis original). As such, it is important to understand how practitioners make use of diagnostic criteria, one example of how practitioners work in line with, around, and in spite of the medical model (Whooley 2010; Schnittker 2017).

Ironically, the forces that influence practitioners to work within the biomedical model can be seen perhaps with the greatest poignancy by looking at those most wedded to psychoanalysis and in-depth talk therapy—those who were historically the least likely to subscribe to a biomedical approach—like Dr. King. Unlike the typical mental health practitioner today, many of the doctors in this study have extensive training in psychoanalysis; investigating their attitudes toward and use of psychopharmacology and diagnosis and understanding how they think about etiology will provide a window into medicalization's reach. Schechter (2014, 14) notes that even psychoanalysts have found ways to adjust to practicing in a field gripped by evidence-based medicine. In her ethnography of psychoanalysis, she notes, as a means of survival, analysts have arrived at "their own opportunistic forms of adaptation to EBM [evidence-based medicine]." How psychoanalysts navigate in a biomedical world is not always predictable, and it affords insight into many of the key issues facing the mental health fields today. How do mental health practitioners with varying training backgrounds operate in a field dominated by evidence-based practices and biomedicine? Psychoanalysts and other mental health practitioners who work outside the biomedical model have had to adapt. At the same time, some of the core principles of psychodynamic psychotherapy—namely the importance of the relationship between the patient and practitioner in the treatment—have not been erased entirely from the landscape of mental health practice. As Metzl (2003, 4) argues, psychopharmacology has not fully eclipsed these basic notions. However, biomedical psychiatry has certainly eroded their consideration, and the time students spend learning how to have therapeutic relationships with their patients has diminished significantly, as curricula focus on diagnosis and medicinal solutions to the range of psychiatric troubles. Perhaps psychodynamic principles will never again be foregrounded in a typical mental health treatment. Yet the practitioners I spoke with were clear that mental health paradigms evolve, often oscillating between more and less biological and psychological paradigms. And in every era when one dominates the field, dissenting voices loom in the background even if they are not always outspoken, and today many call for the integration of various treatment models. What the future of psychiatry and mental health treatment more generally will look like as the twenty-first century carries on is unclear. Some of my interviewees suggest that the dominant ideas in the mental health fields move like a pendulum; although new ideas emerge, they often describe a sense of vacillating back and forth over time. Some describe a more circular trajectory wherein the notion of progress is somewhat elusive. Regardless, most are clear that the biomedical model is here, likely to remain the dominant paradigm; how this plays out in practice and what it means for practitioners to carry out their work under the influence of the biomedical model have until now been less clear.

Overview

Chapter 1—"From Meaning Making to Medicalization"—provides an overview of the biomedical model's rise to dominance in psychiatry and its impact on other mental health professionals. For a paradigm that cannot offer the identification of a physical lesion, as in the case of cancer or arterial disease, the biomedical model has been remarkably successful at shaping notions of etiology and appropriate treatment and relatively swiftly pushed psychoanalysis to the periphery of the field. This chapter provides the historical context in which the practitioners in this study evaluate and treat patients; it is a glimpse into the recent history and general topography of the biomedical world in which they practice as well as the psychodynamic principles that some still employ.

Chapter 2—"Practitioner Portraits and Pathways to Practice"—offers an in-depth look at four practitioners who are characteristic of others with similar training. Specifically, I explore their decisions to become mental health practitioners, what their training trajectories looked like, and how they think about key issues in their field. The themes that emerge in these four portraits, specifically the central role of diagnosis and medication, attitudes toward talk therapy, and challenges presented by the biomedical model, are those I explore in greater depth in the remaining chapters.

Chapter 3—"The Promise of 'Imperfect Communication' and the 'Prison' of Rigid Categorization: The DSM in Practice"—takes a close look at the role of the DSM in practice and how it is involved in practitioners' thinking about patients. Discrete categorization is a central part of mental health treatment, but some practitioners struggle with the rigidity of the manual, and many lament the loss of meaning-making practices and contextualization of patients' life experiences that were once central to the field. Practitioners describe using the DSM because it helps organize their thinking, and it helps them communicate with other practitioners about their patients' symptoms, but some also feel pressure to use it because it allows patients to be reimbursed for their treatment and because it is considered "best practice" to engage in formal diagnosis. Regardless of their attitudes toward the DSM, it anchors practice to the biomedical model and evidence-based medicine.

Chapter 4—"Etiological Considerations and the Tools of the Trade: The Role of Medication and Talk Therapy in Practice"—is about practitioners' conceptualizations of etiology and the connection of those ideas about the derivations of their patients' symptoms with treatment. Practitioners' reliance on and belief in the utility of medications are directly linked to the extent to which they believe their patients' symptoms are born of biology. Furthermore, practitioners who were trained medically (psychiatrists) are more likely than those who were not (psychologists) to feel that being a good doctor involves prescribing medications. There are also significant external forces on practice that make it increasingly likely that my interviewees not only see their patients' conditions as medical problems but also offer medical solutions for them: patients often want medications, insurance companies prefer to pay for medications than for talk therapy, and pharmaceutical companies attempt to pressure practitioners into prescribing certain kinds of medications. I also address the deep belief that many of my interviewees share—that talk therapy can change people's lives and free people from a range of troubles. While the biomedical model often trumps the psychodynamic, talk therapy is still an important part of some practitioners' treatment plans to help people live more satisfying, less conflict-laden lives. Though there is a broad body of research on the role of the DSM in practice, treatment decisions—the reasons practitioners use medication and talk therapy—are much less well understood. In particular, the relationship between how practitioners think about etiology and the kinds of treatments they recommend is important for understanding the impact of training on practice—how and why doctors employ various interventions. In talking about their rationales for treatment, it is also clear that uncertainty about etiology and treatment efficacy is an influential force in practitioners' treatment decisions.

Chapter 5—"The Consequences of the Biomedical Model for Practice and Practitioners: Psychodynamic Therapy in a Biomedical World"—is about the consequences of practicing under the influence of the biomedical model. For practitioners trained largely in psychopharmacology, their work and professional perspective are largely unchallenged. Their credentials and training put them in a position to practice in line with the dominant treatment in the field. Yet all other practitioners describe tensions that take the shape of both internal and interpersonal conflict. For those who practice extensive talk therapy and who are deeply entrenched in thinking about a range of factors from early childhood experiences to current life situations, the use of medication and biological thinking about etiology is more problematic and conflict-laden. Also challenging is practicing in a field ruled by biomedicine without the ability to prescribe medications, which is the case for psychologists. The kinds of conflicts practitioners face offer further insight into how the biomedical model maintains its dominance. This chapter shows how training, which is linked to both literal credentials as well as attitudes toward medication and talk therapy, leads practitioners to experience their field and treatment in different ways.

I conclude with a reflection on how diagnosis, the use of medication, and thinking about etiology not only are representative of medicalization but also propel it forward. My interviewees exist in a medical field, where basic psychodynamic principles are still important but, because of social forces and institutional pressures, cannot have the influence they once did. Furthermore, patients and practitioners alike are less exposed to psychodynamic ideas, which push them to rely more on biomedical notions of etiology and psychopharmacology. Medicalization has settled in, and now practitioners in different camps work with the biomedical model, even when they disagree with some of its most basic assumptions. Some practitioners are optimistic that the principles of psychodynamically informed talk therapy such as transference and the role of the unconscious can remain relevant insofar as they inform the central feature of a treatment: the relationship between the practitioner and the patient. Furthermore, practitioners are aware of what Conrad and Schneider (1980) referred to as the "bright" and "dark" consequences of medicalization. In the 1980s and 1990s, psychopharmacology was still in something of a honeymoon phase, but the practitioners with whom I spoke are clear that there is ambiguity today around the outcomes of psychopharmacology and some concern about the central role of diagnosis. Some hope this will open the door for a renewed interest in non-biomedical forms of treatment, though there is little evidence it will. Given the power of managed care, big pharma, and patient demand, which all work to uphold the biomedical model (Conrad 2005), in combination with cultural models that support biomedical thinking about etiology and treatment, the biomedical model in mental health treatment is likely not at risk of losing its grip. Furthermore, the practitioners in this study, even those who hope for a reintegration of some key psychodynamic principles into mainstream practice, are unlikely to actively resist this advanced state of medicalization—many support it—and all have a hand in perpetuating it.

Chapter 1

From Meaning Making to Medicalization

The biomedical and psychodynamic approaches nurture two very different moral instincts by shaping differently the fundamental categories that are the tools of the ways we reason about our responsibilities in caring for those in pain: who is a person (not an obvious question), what constitutes that person's pain, who are we to intervene, what intervention is good. These two approaches teach their practitioners to look at people differently. They have different contradictions and different bottom lines. Both have their strengths and their weaknesses. Each changes the way doctors perceive patients, the way society perceives patients, and the way patients perceive themselves.

—T. M. Luhrmann, *Of Two Minds*

Over the course of the late twentieth century a radical shift occurred in psychiatry. The *Freudian*, *psychoanalytic*, or *psychodynamic* talking cure that dominated psychiatric (and most mental health) practice ceded prominence to the *biomedical* model.[1] This transformation felt like a paradigm shift. The movement toward evidence-based medicine and neuroscience involved a dismissal (some say a rejection) of most of the central features of the psychodynamic model and seemed to occur almost overnight. In many ways, however, the path toward biomedical psychiatry was a more gradual sea change in which long-lurking bio-medical theories and treatments regained prominence in the field. Regardless, palpable contention characterized the field of psychiatry in the late twentieth century as practitioners battled for the future of a field now overwhelmingly under the influence of the biomedical model. There is no doubt that by the 1980s biological thinking and a focus on diagnosis transported psychiatry from a dis-cipline that valued deep exploration of the psyche to one that advocates short-term, biomedical treatments.

While the history of late twentieth-century psychiatry is far too extensive to explore here and has been expertly recounted elsewhere (see especially Decker 2013; Horwitz 2002a; Shorter 1993), I address in the following pages the background for the conditions under which the doctors in this study practice. As such, I offer a glimpse into psychiatry in the psychoanalytic era and a brief foray into the story of how mental health troubles came under the purview of the biomedical model, with a focus on key ideas, principles of practice, and his-torical moments in each paradigm. Even more swiftly than it rose to prominence, the psychodynamic tradition—anchored in exploration of the relationship between analyst and analysand (patient), understanding of the unconscious, conflict and defense, and examination of the impact of early experience on the evolving personality—was relegated to the periphery of the field. The biomedi-cal model in psychiatry is now settled and is the overarching framework within which mental health practitioners operate. In particular, psychiatrists today are mostly trained to diagnose discrete symptoms as mental disorder using the clas-sificatory system detailed in the *Diagnostic and Statistical Manual of Mental Disorders* (DSM) and to prescribe medications as treatment for what are seen as heritable conditions based in neurobiology. This chapter focuses largely on psychiatry, although this story is relevant to other mental health fields, given psychiatry's wide-ranging influence over diagnostic and treatment standards. Furthermore, the same forces that ushered in biomedical psychiatry—managed care, pharmaceuticals, evidence-based medicine, and shifting consumer desires—broadly impact mental health practitioners.

The Psychoanalytic Heyday: Exploration of the Psyche and the Meaning of Symptoms

Medical historian Roy Porter (1997, 516) describes Freudian psychoanalysis as having "changed the self-image of the western mind." Though the psychoanalytic heyday was but a "hiatus" between early and current biological models (Shorter 1997), once psychiatry was awash in psychoanalytic principles, neither the field nor broader notions of the psyche and the self would be the same. Freud published *The Interpretation of Dreams* in 1900 and made his only trip to the United States in 1909 (to deliver a keynote speech at Clark University), yet his work didn't influence American psychiatry until the 1920s and was not widely read until around 1940, one year after his death (Hale 1995; Lunbeck 1994). Freud's ideas posthumously revolutionized American psychiatry and conceptualizations of mental illness more broadly, and by the 1950s both were firmly psychodynamic.

In post–World War II American culture, increasing secularism and social conservatism (especially surrounding sexuality) made for fertile ground in which psychoanalysis could take root. Combined with the rising antipsychiatry movement, the notion that therapeutic relationships could alleviate symptoms fueled a desire for a more humanistic way of understanding illness and the mind in general. The psychodynamic approach countered the biological thinking that dominated American psychiatry in the early 1900s, when the prevailing theories depicted mental illness as a brain disorder, which allowed for crude practices like lobotomy and primitive forms of electroconvulsive therapy, among other experimental practices, to be used regularly, with the goal of altering the physical properties of the brain.[2] People who experienced psychiatric troubles were set apart from other members of society, often via isolation in state psychiatric facilities. Based on the notion that mental illness was not a drastically different state of being from normality, psychoanalytic theory presented a new language for understanding psychiatric conditions.

For Freud, good mental health was dependent on successful resolution of early psychosexual stages of development. Both dysfunction and healthier outcomes potentially emerged from progression through these universal stages; the latter were seen as proceeding in a biologically dictated order (oral, anal, phallic, etc.), but forward development could be derailed by the possible interplay of both external factors (e.g., trauma, overstimulation, deprivation, etc.) and internal dynamics (e.g., intense conflict over unconscious wishes). Mental life was viewed as dynamic, reflecting an ever-changing, active relationship between reality and mental forces, potentially leading to guilt, conflict, and symptom formation (Greenson 1995; Brenner 1974).

Freud conceptualized most of his patients' symptoms as representing a *neurosis*;[3] the creation of overt symptoms, designed to mask forbidden unconscious emotions and fantasies, was believed to protect the patient from the overwhelming anxiety that would result from emergence of such material into conscious awareness. This was the central concern of Freudian psychoanalysis (Brenner 1974). Neuroses were presumed to be the result of early psychic conflicts, rooted in psychological mechanisms such as fantasies and wishes, rather than purely in biological malfunctioning. Psychoanalysis was oriented toward the influence of past psychological conflicts on the present, and the assumption that the mind is ever changing, active, in motion—in short, a constant dynamic interplay between reality and mental forces, potentially leading to conflict and possibly to symptom formation. Problems, namely neurotic symptoms, emerged from conflictual wishes during childhood psychosexual stages. One could become "fixated" or stuck in a particular stage (e.g., the oral stage) and later develop a neurotic tendency in that vein (e.g., nail biting). These deviations could happen to anyone, as no one navigates childhood development entirely unscathed. Freudian psychiatry diminished the exoticism of psychiatric troubles by reconceptualizing them as inevitable reaction to the ubiquitous conflicts, wishes, and fantasies that arise in relation to everyday childhood experiences or trauma. In this way, Freudian theory was both universalist (everyone must go through these stages) and individualist (patients navigated these stages in unique ways). Freud conceptualized more severe psychiatric conditions, *psychosis*, on a continuum with neurotic symptoms, thus making their sufferers seem less worthy of the isolation of asylum settings. Yet because neurotic symptoms were more directly in the wheelhouse of psychoanalytic treatment, psychoanalysis shifted the attention of psychiatrists and laypeople alike away from psychotic illnesses like schizophrenia, which had been the focus of psychiatry through the early twentieth century (Porter 1997).

As a treatment, psychoanalysis sought to mitigate the influence of past psychological conflicts on present functioning. Targeting mostly patients with neurotic symptoms, the Freudian approach helped analysands situate their symptoms in a biographical context with the idea that examination of the patient's verbal processes and reactions to the analyst could lead to recognition of unconscious conflicts and past (especially repressed) emotions and experiences. Over an extended period of time, the patient's free associations and reactions to the analyst, in combination with the analyst's interpretations of hidden fantasies, relational patterns, and defensive mechanisms, would lead to insight about unconscious processes; ultimately, new ways of thinking and experiencing self and others were expected to free people from their neurotic tendencies, whether phobias of insects or sexual inhibitions. In short, for Freudians, the gradual exploration and restructuring of ever-changing subconscious processes—present in all human beings at all times and within the context of the patient-analyst relationship—is the basis of psychoanalytic treatment. Establishing connections between present thought and behavior, unconscious processes required deep knowledge of patients, which was gained in extensive, in-depth treatment usually involving four to five sessions per week. The complexity of psychoanalysis is exemplified by longitudinal case studies that provide detailed information about individual patients' life stories, character, and personality, as illustrated by Freud's "Ratman," "Wolfman," and "Little Hans" (Freud [1940] 2003). The goal for the analysand, as described by the science writer Morton Hunt in his opus on the history of psychology, was "an awareness of one's unconscious motives and the attainment of a state in which choices were determined by conscious ones" (1993, 186).

The Freudian model, already well established in Europe (with both fervent challengers and devout followers), rose to prominence in the United States because of a number of key figures in American psychoanalysis, perhaps most importantly Harry Stack Sullivan (Greenberg and Mitchell 1983). Freud's contemporaries were divided as to what extent psychoanalysts should take culture into consideration when treating patients. Sullivan advocated for and advanced psychoanalytic techniques, but also vehemently disagreed with the lack of context in Freud's drive theory.[4] Most importantly, Sullivan pointed to an "underemphasis [of] the larger social and cultural context," which, he argued, "must figure prominently in any theory attempting to account for the origins, development, and warpings of personality" (Greenberg and Mitchell 1983, 80). Sullivan's work was heavily influenced by the pragmatist school, of which he was well informed during his years at the University of Chicago by both psychiatrists and social theorists such as George Herbert Mead, Charles H. Cooley, and Robert Park. An investigation of macro-social influences on individual-level phenomena abounded in the work of these theorists, who suggested that social structures were key factors in determining people's life chances. There was, therefore, a deeply social bent to Sullivan's work, especially in his focus on how interaction and relationships affected psychological function and troubles.

Sullivan's attention to culture and context is a prime example of the deep divide between American psychoanalysts and early Biomedical Psychiatrists. Because Sullivan studied in the 1920s, he was familiar with American asylums at their peak. He spent much of his career studying schizophrenia, since the severe symptoms of this disorder (namely hallucinations and delusions) were likely to lead to treatment in institutional settings. At the time, Emil Kraepelin's biological theory of schizophrenia dominated thinking in the field. Responsible for many of the earliest classifications of mental illness, Kraepelin is both lauded and denounced for his conceptualizations and measurements of specific mental illness categories with discrete symptom sets (Decker 2013; Horwitz

2002a; Kirk and Kutchins 1992). The Kraepelinian model made it more manageable to identify and treat patients' symptoms. Many, including Sullivan, however, became critical of the Kraepelinian classification scheme; Sullivan went as far as to claim that the Kraepelinian approach was more about the researcher's attempt to objectify and characterize the patient than to understand or make sense of the patient's behavior.[5] American psychiatry was fraught with debate between those in favor of discrete, rigid classification and those who supported a focus on experience and context, and much of this is echoed in debates about the perils and promise of the biomedical model that dominate psychiatry today.

A force in establishing the prominence of psychoanalysis in American psychiatry, Sullivan became one of the founding theorists and practitioners of American psychodynamic psychiatry. It is in great part due to his efforts that dynamic psychiatry was infused with such a strong opposition to the biomedical approach and that many American psychoanalysts were so concerned with interpersonal relationships. Sullivan was a powerful figure and successfully pushed psychiatrists to avoid conceptualizations of psychiatric symptoms as representations of biological malfunctioning. Though many early analysts were medical doctors, there was a heavier reliance on philosophy and theories of the mind than on diagnosis and biology; key figures in analysis were well trained in the philosophy of science and hoped to further their discipline by advancing theories on the etiology of mental disorders (Greenberg and Mitchell 1983). The emphasis on patients' experiences was in line with the broader practice of American medicine. Psychoanalysis emerged during an era in which doctors had ongoing relationships with patients, as managed care had not yet impacted the doctor-patient relationship (Porter 1997). Though psychiatry has always been concerned with some form of diagnosis, psychiatrists in the 1950s and 1960s were rarely preoccupied with discrete classification. In the psychodynamic tradition, symptoms were a starting point but were located in the context of patients' complex lives.

While illness classification manuals, such as the DSM, play a central role in psychiatry today, practitioners rarely consulted such manuals in the psychodynamic era (Kirk and Kutchins 1992). Even though DSM-II, the edition available for use from the 1960s until 1980, was written from a psychodynamic perspective, it was largely irrelevant to psychiatric practice, as illness categories in classic psychoanalysis were vague and not meant for acute diagnosis. DSM-II was divided into "neurotic" and "psychotic" categories, unmistakably Freudian terminology.[6] One of a small number of conditions under the heading "neuroses, anxiety neuroses" was described in the following manner: "This neurosis is characterized by anxious over-concern extending to panic and frequently associated with somatic symptoms. Unlike *phobic neurosis* [a second neurotic category] . . . anxiety may occur under any circumstances and is not restricted to specific situations or objects. This disorder must be distinguished from normal apprehension or fear, which occurs in realistically dangerous situations" (APA 1968). DSM-II provided a vague, general outline of a condition, without a specific description of symptoms for identifying a disorder; the practitioner was responsible for contextualizing symptoms based on an intimate knowledge of the patient. Even though dynamic psychiatrists recorded symptoms, they were not concerned with objective classification. Light (1980, 180) aptly captures the dynamic tradition when he describes practitioners who search for "'clues' to the patient's dynamics." Psychiatrists sought to uncover how patients think and how past conditions affect present experiences, which meant discrete diagnosis was largely irrelevant.

Dynamic psychiatry revolutionized the way people viewed mental illness and provided society with a language and a forum for talking about and questioning the concept of abnormality. The spread of dynamic psychiatry was in no small part due to the emergence of what Horwitz (2002a) calls a "culture of psychotherapy." This culture, however, depended on individuals who were educated and had ample incomes. Dynamic psychiatry offered freedom from repression, which was particularly appealing given post–World War II political and social conservatism, especially pertaining to sexuality. Jewish Americans, sexual minorities, and other oppressed groups were especially interested in the idea of psychological exploration, and artists, writers, and academics routinely sought the help of analysts for everything from difficulty with work and relationships to severe symptoms of depression. Despite its having been the dominant theoretical and treatment paradigm for but a moment, psychodynamic psychiatry had an immense impact on the mental health professions, and it flourished in the United States in the mid-1900s because of a pool of patients interested in and with the resources to afford its intensive treatment, as well as a range of cultural conditions that fostered an openness to its brand of treatment.

Enter the Biomedical Model

As the prevailing American political and social epistemologies shifted in the latter part of the twentieth century, psychodynamic psychiatry lost its foothold as the dominant means for dealing with psychological distress. The belief in the importance of "hard science," grounded in facts and proof, became increasingly important to all scientific disciplines, especially psychiatry, which was struggling to be seen as a legitimate medical field. Psychoanalysis was ill equipped to defend against accusations that it was an unscientific means for dealing with illness, as its entire basis was in interpretation (Hale 1995, 300–301; Horwitz 2002a); the lack of demonstrable validity and reliability in case analysis left psychoanalysis open to criticism and increasing calls for a new classification system (Kirk and Kutchins 1992, 28–32). The critics were increasingly vocal by the 1970s. As early as 1966, prominent psychiatrist Lawrence Kubie had noted deep divisions between his colleagues: "Some are so dedicated to the organic approach that they are terrified lest their fragment of truth not contain all the answers and they thereby be lost. Out of such terror come furious and poison-penned attacks on all psychological considerations and methods. The same terror assails some of those who approach psychiatric disorders from an exclusively psychological basis. They too live in terror lest a drug come along to destroy their life's work and hopes; and they too react with rage" (Falck 1980, 223). Acknowledging vehement opposition between Freudian psychoanalysts and those wedded to the biological approach—who even then were urging the psychodynamically dominated field to think more biologically—he referred to psychoanalysts as "organophobic" (fearful of organic, biological thinking) and identified the emerging voices in favor of medications and diagnostic thinking as "psychophobic" (afraid of any validity to the psychoanalytic tradition).

Popular culture jabbed at the increasing doubts about the efficacy of psychoanalysis, as epitomized by Alvy Singer, the protagonist of Woody Allen's 1977 film *Annie Hall*. The demonstrably neurotic Singer pointed out that he had been in analysis for fifteen years. By the 1970s, psychiatry floundered in the face of deinstitutionalization, the emergence of new medications, and the rising power of managed care.[7] Psychoanalysis came to be seen as an unscientific, subjective means of dealing with illness. Facing a wave of structural demands for efficiency it could not withstand, it was out of seeming necessity and a new allegiance to biomedicine that psychiatry shifted toward a more evidence-based model. Especially with a population of formerly institutionalized people thrust into community settings, the promise of efficient treatment with measurable efficacy was desirable and necessary (Hale 1995; Horwitz 2002a; Shorter 1993, 1998). Some psychoanalysts realized their methods were not amenable to the treatment of individuals with severe mental illnesses, though Freud and his colleagues did (controversially) treat a handful of patients with quite severe psychotic symptoms.

Many classically trained psychoanalysts were adamantly opposed to measuring the effectiveness of their treatments and the progress of their patients using quantifiable measures. An evidence-based model was counterintuitive to the way they conceptualized the psyche and psychiatric treatment; however, their resistance to empirical approaches came to be seen as a marker of the rigidity of psychoanalysts and the dogmatism of psychoanalysis, critiques still levied today (McWilliams 2000, 375). Consider an interchange between Peter Rudnytsky, author of many volumes on psychoanalysis, and Roy Schafer, a prominent and classically trained psychoanalyst. Rudnytsky interviewed Schafer in 2000, when Schafer was in his eighties. Rudnytsky mentions a famous psychoanalytic study of children, noting, "Empirical studies seem to me to play an indispensable role in sifting out which theories in psychoanalysis continue to be vital and which theories are outmoded." Schafer responds with a resounding "no," pushing Rudnytsky to question "whether psychoanalytic theory, either of a particular school or considered as a totality, is something that can be assessed within any framework outside that of psychoanalysis itself, or can it find its validation only from within its own way of thinking?" Schafer responds, "That's what I believe . . . I object to its being called a science" (Rudnytsky 2000, 225–226). Some analysts, well into the biomedical era in psychiatry, refused to think of their discipline in empirical terms; psychoanalysis was out of step not only with psychiatry, but with American medicine more broadly, which had rapidly become focused on evidence-based medicine. Existential wonderings, interpretations of meaning, questions of human nature, and individual-oriented treatments were increasingly unacceptable; a treatment approach was no longer scientific if it could not be held accountable for its effectiveness (Porter 1997 Starr 1982).

Because of its basis in a set of strict diagnostic criteria, biomedical psychiatry offered a strategy for measuring progress much more clearly than was possible with talk therapy. Scientific inquiry, equated with objectivity, led to an increased call for proof of efficacy, and psychoanalysis was simply not a discipline set up to measure progress in quantifiable terms (Shorter 1993, 1998). As Horwitz (2002a, 5–6) explains, "For its advocates, the model of mental illness in diagnostic psychiatry is not just different from, but better than the earlier dynamic model because the scientific methods it employs are equated with objectivity, truth, and reason." The biomedical model, equated with hard science and empiricism, came to be seen as the valid brand of psychiatry (Hale 1995; Horwitz 2002a; Shorter 1998). Emblematic of the quest for validity and reliability was the publication of DSM-III in 1980. Chaired by Columbia University's Robert Spitzer (retired professor of psychiatry at Columbia University and chief of the Biometrics Research Department at the New York State Psychiatric Institute) and including many other biologically minded psychiatrists, the taskforce for the new manual was oriented toward categorical thinking. Unlike the broad categories in DSM-II, DSM-III shifted the focus of psychiatry to pathology.[8] DSM-III (and its more recent counterparts, DSM-III-R, IV, IV-TR, and 5) classified illness entities that are identified based on particular symptoms, which are the focus of treatment.

The release of DSM-III is widely described as a watershed moment in twentieth-century psychiatry (e.g., Horwitz 2002a; Shorter 1998). Gerald Maxmen, author of the popular book *The New Psychiatrists*, unequivocally attributes what he calls "the ascendance of scientific psychiatry" to the DSM-III: "By adopting the scientifically based DSM-III as its official system of diagnosis, American psychiatrists broke with a fifty year tradition of using psychoanalytically based diagnoses. Perhaps more than any other single event, the publication of DSM-III demonstrated that American Psychiatry has indeed undergone a revolution" (quoted in Kirk and Kutchins 1992, 7, 31). Using the language of political upheaval, Maxmen and others noted the momentousness of the new DSM. For Biomedical Psychiatrists, DSM-III represented an exciting potential for psychiatry to reshape its image—to be a true science. At the annual conference of the American Psychiatric Association in 1982, Gerald Klerman, then chief of the Federal Mental Health Agency, the most powerful psychiatrist in the American government, addressed critics of DSM-III: "The theme of this meeting is 'science in the service of healing.' In my opinion, DSM III embodies this theme to a greater extent than any other achievement in American psychiatry since the advent of the new drugs" (quoted in Kirk and Kutchins 1992, 6). The biomedical model propelled forth by the new diagnostic system had indeed taken a place of prominence in psychiatry by the 1980s, and reignited the old tensions between biomedically and psychologically oriented psychiatrists that permeated psychiatry throughout the twentieth century.

Characteristic of this move toward symptom sets and discrete categorizations is the radical change in the conceptualization of anxiety. The DSM-III (and its more recent counterparts) classifies disease entities that can be identified based on particular symptoms that represent various types of pathology or abnormality. The DSM-III removed the term "neurosis" from the manual, striking both a figurative and literal blow at psychoanalysis (Shorter 1997). Many of what were neurotic conditions in the era of DSM-II were now considered to be separate disease entities, evidenced by the categorizations of various anxiety disorders e.g. panic disorder, social phobia, simple phobia, obsessive-compulsive disorder, posttraumatic stress disorder, and generalized anxiety disorder. Consider, for instance,

Diagnostic Criteria for Panic Disorder:

A. At least three panic attacks within a three-week period in circumstances other than during marked physical exertion or in a life-threatening situation. The attacks are not precipitated only by exposure to a circumscribed phobic stimulus.

B. Panic attacks are manifested by discrete periods of apprehension or fear, and at least four of the following symptoms appear during each attack:

    1. dyspnea

    2. palpitations

    3. chest pain or discomfort

    4. choking or smothering sensations

    5. dizziness, vertigo, or unsteady feelings

    6. feelings of unreality

    7. paresthesia (tingling in hands or feet)

    8. hot and cold flashes

    9. sweating

    10. faintness

    11. trembling or shaking

    12. fear of dying, going crazy, or doing something uncontrolled during an attack

C. Not due to a physical disorder or another mental disorder, such as major depression, somatization disorder, or schizophrenia.

D. The disorder is not associated with agoraphobia (APA 1987, 231–232)

DSM-III diagnoses classified specific symptom sets. The detailed diagnostic framework for panic disorder, above, accomplishes three crucial tasks at the heart of the biomedical model: first, it distinguishes panic disorder from other kinds of anxiety disorders (point C and D); second, it defines the duration of symptoms necessary for a diagnosis (point A); and third, it identifies the specific symptoms, which assess the severity of the condition (points A and B).

DSM-III provided for psychiatry the same kind of threshold measurement used in other branches of medicine, which seek to identify not only disease itself, but also risk factors for its potential future development. Greene (2007) explains the movement in medicine at large toward diagnosing what were formerly subthreshold diagnoses: "By the close of the 20th Century . . . the diagnosis of any of these conditions required only numerical measurement above a statistically defined threshold. A blood pressure higher than 130/80 mm Hg was now hypertension. A blood LDL . . . cholesterol level greater than 160 mg/dL was pathologically elevated. . . . These numbers are now central to the practice of diagnosis, their precision and standardizability allowing for a definition of disease in which the physical perceptions of doctor and patient are irrelevant" (7–8). If psychiatry was to be seen as evidence-based practice, the DSM was crucial. Unlike in cardiology or oncology, there are no lesions to uncover, no "pathognomonic sign" (Greene 2007, 8). In psychiatry, the discernment of disease relies entirely on identifying symptomatology.[9]

The diagnostic model significantly altered psychiatric training. With the release of DSM-III, interns and residents in psychiatry were expected to learn the new diagnostic categories. As the anthropologist T. M. Luhrmann (2001, 36) observed in her ethnography of psychiatric training, "By the time young psychiatrists have finished training they can recognize the disorders immediately, the way plane spotters can spot Boeing 747s, the way bird-watchers can spot great snowy owls, the way dog lovers know the difference between a Jack Russell terrier and a beagle." In medicine writ large, Jutel (2011, 23) explains, "diagnosis continues to be at the heart of medical education, serving both as objective and heuristic. . . . Disease principles and specific diseases organize how medical students learn about the body." For treating mental health troubles, the DSM is a useful tool for young practitioners, as it provides a clear framework for understanding patients' often confusing symptoms, thus making it easier to enact a treatment plan. Residents may find that mastering diagnosis marks them as professionals with high status in their field (Timmermans and Berg 2003a, 17). Yet, as they are socialized into the discourse and practice of their field, psychiatry residents are rarely taught that the diagnostic method is one possibility in a range of treatment forms; instead, they are instructed that the biomedical model is *the* means for treating illness (Smith and Hemler 2014). And the salience of the DSM model leads to a narrow view of what illness and treatment are, as Light (1980, 160) explains: "Learning how to diagnose is a skill which psychiatric residents must learn before all others. . . . Paradoxically, however, as residents become more seasoned practitioners, diagnosis no longer retains this preeminent role; one learns to formulate a plan of treatment more by feel and common sense. But this may be no paradox at all if 'feel and common sense' have by that time become imbued with the psychiatric mode of diagnosis." The diagnostic categories are so much a part of the psychiatric worldview that they are internalized by practitioners, who feel as though they are classifying natural, objectively observable phenomena. As such, Timmermans and Berg (2003a, 163) observe, one of the crucial roles of more senior clinicians is to offer perspective to their interns and residents as they assess patients precisely because

medical standards are not sufficient and cannot substitute for experience. Nonetheless, the DSM offers a connection to evidence-based medicine in a discipline whose Freudian legacy was ridiculed by other medical fields (and even
from within its own) for its lack of demonstrable validity.

In the 1980s, narrative accounts of psychiatry training depicted a field
divided, but one in which biological thinking was already winning out. Consider the following interaction between a residency supervisor and then psychiatry resident Robert Klitzman (1995, 76) about a patient:

Klitzman: She says she's depressed.
Supervisor: That's not enough for a diagnosis.
Klitzman: She looks kind of depressed, too.
Supervisor: Lots of people say they're depressed, but if she doesn't meet these
    criteria, we don't have target symptoms to follow for marking her progress
    and if we don't it's not worth treating her . . . remember to always DSM-
    III-R your patients in the beginning.

Klitzman (70) recounts receiving competing advice from a psychodynamic psychiatrist, who urged him to learn more about the patient's life. Klitzman
described this as prototypical of his experience in a prominent psychiatry residency program in the 1980s, when residents were often bounced like ping-pong
balls between supervisors wedded to different diagnostic approaches and treatment models.

Perhaps the most significant consequence of training in discrete diagnosis
is that it fosters a loss of attention to nuance and the context of patients' lives,
as Kleinman (1988, 17) notes in his depiction of how psychiatrists trained in
the biomedical model approach patients: "The tale of complaints becomes the
text that is to be decoded by the practitioner cum diagnostician. Practitioners,
however, are not trained to be self-reflective interpreters of distinctive systems
of meaning. They are turned out of medical schools as naïve realists . . . who
are led to believe that symptoms are clues to disease, evidence of a 'natural' process, a physical entity to be discovered or uncovered." This is a dramatic
departure from the philosophically and psychologically oriented practitioner
of the pre-DSM-III era. Luhrmann (2001, 68) articulately summarizes a key distinction, when she explains that, in the biomedical model, "the person diagnosing learns to distill a diagnosis out of a patient's narrative and to see that
many different lives share a common label." In psychodynamic training, however, she says, "the models are rarely taught and memorized abstractly. For the

most part, the models remain specific, as something some patient did at some time that is kind of like what she did some months later." In the diagnostic tradition psychiatrists are not concerned with the case-specific elements of the patient's experience. In fact, they are trained not to be. A psychodynamic practice, conversely, leaves practitioners with case-specific information, much of which is so intimately related to the individual patient that it cannot be generalized. Though this was seen as a strength in the eyes of many psychodynamic practitioners, this idiographic view of patients as unique, subjective beings was seen as a weakness of the psychoanalytic model in the late twentieth century.

DSM-III also had significant consequences for the conceptualization of symptoms, particularly in terms of the severity of illness. The discrete and exhaustive categories lowered the threshold for diagnosis; many formerly sub-threshold symptoms that were seen as natural parts of life or normal distress were now considered pathological (Horwitz 2002a, 2002b; Horwitz and Wakefield 2007). As such, DSM-III can be described as an instrument of medicalization—it classifies much of human experience as medical disorder (Conrad 1992, 211). Psychiatry, mirroring medicine at large, aided in the expansion of what Greene (2007, 4) calls "the domain of chronic diseases." DSM-III classification led to an inflation of the number of people who were seen as disordered, increasing the potential pool of patients, which set the stage for pharmaceutical companies to target patients with specific DSM diagnoses for particular medications. Critics worried that the new psychiatry promoted, for psychiatrists and patients alike, what Porter (1997, 718) called the "fantasy that everyone has something wrong with them, everyone and everything can be cured."

The cure took the form of psychotropic medications. As early as the 1960s, but especially in the 1970s and 1980s, clinical trials gained prominence in medical research as a central tool of the biomedical model (Horwitz 2002a; Porter 1997; Starr 1982). In the 1980s, pharmaceutical companies released and psychiatrists began to widely prescribe a new kind of so-called antidepressants.[10] In 1987 the FDA approved the use of Prozac, a selective serotonin reuptake inhibitor (SSRI), which claimed to selectively target the neurotransmitter serotonin (a key neurotransmitter thought to be responsible for depression and anxiety, the two most widely diagnosed psychiatric troubles). Marketed as safe and effective compared to older classes of antidepressants and antianxiety medications, Prozac ushered in the era of psychotropic medications. In the 1990s, pharmaceutical companies released a range of new SSRIs in the mold of Eli Lilly's Prozac, which the psychiatrist Peter Kramer (1993) famously described as having the potential to reveal the true self and to make people feel better than well. The broad excitement about SSRIs ushered in an era of widespread medication use for depression and anxiety, which (with the exception of antianxiety agents in the 1950s) had been used much more sparingly in the past. Much as they rejected DSM-III categorizations, many psychoanalysts staunchly opposed the widespread use of psychopharmacology. Some not only refused to prescribe medications, but would not even see patients who were taking psychotropic medications at all.

By 1994, Prozac was already atop the list of best-selling drugs in the United States and aided in the reification of the conditions listed in the DSM (Shorter 1998, 324); Prozac appeared to the general public to be effective at treating the DSM symptoms of depression, and psychiatrists were optimistic about the prospect of safe, effective treatment for the most common psychiatric symptoms. Yet the evidence in clinical trials was mixed at best, mostly pointing to little improvement over older medications (Grob and Horwitz 2010). When it comes to depression, the most commonly diagnosed mental disorder of the twenty-first century, SSRIs perform relatively poorly in clinical trials, particularly for mild and moderate conditions, and demonstrate even worse efficacy in longitudinal follow-up studies than in short clinical trials (Moncrieff and Kirsch 2005). Furthermore, argue Grob and Horwitz (2010 138), "The relative responsiveness to drugs might have even more to do with differential temperament or personality as opposed to the nature of the symptoms that individuals display." Questions about the dangers associated with SSRIs also remained opaque, and some clinicians and researchers suggested there was a significant risk of suicide (especially for teenagers) associated with the medications and of dependency (Healy 2004). Despite extensive research that demonstrated little merit for the serotonin theory of depression, psychiatry continued to support the wide use of SSRIs (Whitaker 2002, 72–73) and pharmaceutical companies persisted in mass producing and marketing the drugs to the general public. They were able to do so successfully especially once the FDA approved the use of direct-to-consumer advertising in 1998, which reinforced the link between medications and specific DSM diagnoses by leading patients to conceptualize their problems in the language of DSM disorders and to present them as such to physicians (Rose 2006, 478–479).

The notion that biology underlay the array of psychiatric troubles was the foundation for the belief that medications were the appropriate treatment. The fundamental theories in psychiatry regarding etiology shifted, especially as brain scanning technologies and neuroscience became more central to the field.[11] Mental illness was now viewed as biologically born and chemically driven. As Horwitz (2002a, 57) succinctly explains, diagnostic psychiatry "regards diseases as natural entities that exist in the body and that generate the particular symptoms a person displays." Yet the DSM claims no explicit etiological assumptions. In recognizing the mixed evidence for biological etiology, DSM-III claimed to be descriptive, but "generally atheoretical with regard to etiology." Subsequent iterations of the DSM maintained a similar proclamation. Consider this paragraph from the introduction to DSM-IV-TR, in which the APA (2000, xxxiii) cautions use of the DSM in forensic work precisely because it wants to make no etiological claims or assumptions about implications: "A diagnosis does not carry any necessary implications regarding the causes of the individual's mental disorder or its associated impairments. Inclusion of a disorder in the Classification (as in medicine generally) does not require that there be knowledge about its etiology. Moreover, the fact that an individual's presentation meets the criteria for a DSM-IV diagnosis does not carry any necessary implication regarding the individual's degree of control over the behaviors that may be associated with the disorder." In addition, DSM-5 (APA 2013, 25) includes the caveat that "a diagnosis does not carry any necessary implications regarding etiology or causes of the individual's mental disorder or the individual's degree of control over the behaviors that may be associated with the disorder." One significant change in DSM-5 is the creeping notion of biological etiology. In describing mental disorders, DSM-5 mentions the potential impact of "shared genetic and environmental risk factors, and shared neural substrates" (APA 2013, 6). One reason for this longtime noncommittal identification with biological theories of etiology is limited evidence.

The exact mechanism of the biological etiology of mental illness is unclear at best and is described as such, even in widely used psychiatry textbooks. Consider Hyman and Nestler's (2005, 173) portrayal of the uncertainty around genetic etiology: "Vulnerability to many of the most severe psychiatric disorders appears to be heritable, and identification of the specific genes and proteins involved would similarly revolutionize the practice of psychiatry. However, despite great effort, at the time of this writing, it has not yet been possible to identify the specific genes responsible for mental disorders." As such, Schnittker (2017, 219) argues, "the mind-brain connection is as much an issue of philosophy as it is of science." Yet the biomedical model itself leads to a belief in biological causation, and the presumed efficacy of medications offers a teleological explanation that biology, neurochemistry, and heritability are responsible for the range of conditions from depression to schizophrenia.

Despite the DSM's vague stance on etiology and the limited evidence in support of neural substrates, the biomedical paradigm is concerned with disorders of the brain, which produce symptoms that are identified in systematic ways and treated with medication—often, as Cassell (2004) argues, as both the means of and the end to a treatment. Biomedical psychiatry reconceptualized as organic illness conditions what were, in the dynamic tradition, considered a basic part of the human psyche (Horwitz 2002a, 68). Mental pain and suffering became diagnosable and located in the physical brain, and therefore treated with alterations in the chemical culprits. Gilman (1987, 312) and others described the DSM-centric approach as a "re-Kraepelinization of American Psychiatry." Rogler (1997) similarly depicts the biomedical turn as a "remedicalization" of psychiatry, suggesting that the move to biomedical psychiatry is not a new stage but a step backward toward pre-Freudian theories of illness—as if to wipe the slate clean of the psychodynamic approach (particularly true of DSM-III and DSM-5).

The DSM was also a tool applauded by insurance companies in their attempts to manage psychiatric care and cut the costs of treatment. The emergence of managed care was one of the most influential factors that pressured both doctors and patients into short-term, evidence-based treatments—and away from in-depth talk therapy. Psychoanalyst Nancy McWilliams (2000, 373) eloquently describes the denigration of psychoanalysis and the perilous state of psychodynamically informed talk therapy today:

> In the United States, the voice of the individual practitioner is no match for corporate forces. Managed care organizations, whose focus on the bottom line demands promulgating the myth that long-term therapies are ineffective, brand psychoanalytic approaches as empirically unsupported and productive of an unhealthy dependency. Disturbing adaptations to market forces corrupt the very definition of psychotherapy, as HMOs insist that a couple of sessions with a provider willing to sit on their panels and comply with their profit-driven restrictions constitutes the standard of care. . . . The public, although increasingly upset about managed care in general, is still largely ignorant about the magnitude of erosion in their psychotherapy coverage. Even when it is widely known that good mental health care is impossible under the terms of many insurance plans, the stigma associated with psychological disabilities discourages all but the bravest from imploring our union representatives or employers for better mental health benefits.

Clinical practice guidelines—first from government agencies and then from the American Psychiatric Association—were highly influential in pushing practitioners to focus on efficiency and cost effectiveness even before managed care (Barlow 1996, 1050–1051). Practitioners who did not follow these guidelines did so at their own peril. For instance, they were not protected against malpractice suits. These guidelines, which encourage pharmacological treatment and generally downplay the effectiveness of talk therapy, emerged first for depression and not long after for many other illnesses, such as eating disorders, substance abuse, and bipolar disorder. Powerful lobbying groups such as NAMI (National Alliance for Mental Illness) also pushed for the legitimacy of the biomedical model, largely as a way to decrease stigma, but also because the identification of a condition as biological marks it as a real medical entity, one insurance companies are more likely to reimburse.

Finally, marshaling the biomedical model protected the professional dominance of psychiatrists in the field of mental health. The psychodynamic model had opened the door for psychologists, social workers, and even laymen to engage in talking cure treatments (Kirk and Kutchins 1992, 8). By the release of DSM-III, nonmedical mental health practitioners provided equal rates of outpatient treatment as psychiatrists; one-third of treatment was by psychiatrists, another third by psychologists, and the last third by social workers (Hale 1995, 340). Yet only psychiatrists can prescribe medication, the central tool of the biomedical model in psychiatry, which renders its dominance advantageous for the profession. Practitioners from outside of psychiatry have moved in on what Strauss and colleagues (1981, 368) described as the "province of mental health, which has been defined so far as the province of psychiatry, a branch of medicine," yet no other mental health professional can prescribe medications. Medication treatment is what keeps psychiatrists at the top of the hierarchy. Even if many non–medically trained practitioners practice more in-depth talk therapy than psychiatrists, the dominance of the biomedical model combined with psychiatrists' unique ability to prescribe medications allows them to retain power in the field. Kirk and Kutchins (1992, 8) explain that DSM-III, which lays out the criteria upon which medical treatment is based, was created at least partly in order "to reverse diffusion of power to other professions in the mental health enterprise."

Taken together, these powerful influences led to a psychiatric community that widely accepted the biomedical model and largely supported its ascendancy by adopting a diagnostic model and favoring treatment with psychotropic medications.[12] In-depth talk therapy now occupies a peripheral status in mainstream psychiatric treatment. By 1990 the face of psychiatry had changed dramatically, as Hale (1995, 302) explains: "At top ten medical schools only three chairmen were psychoanalysts or members of psychoanalytic organizations. . . . [The] orientation of clinical psychologists . . . also changed; where 41 percent saw themselves as 'psychodynamic' in 1961, by 1976 this had dropped to 19 percent." And by the time DSM-5 arrived in 2013, the diagnostic model swallowed up personality disorders, the last remaining vestige of Freudian language in the DSM. Personality disorders were a distinct set of conditions until DSM-5; the manual divided them into Axis I (largely mood and thought) and Axis II (personality) disorders. The latter was the expertise of psychoanalysts who often specialized in treating narcissism and borderline personality, for example.

Prescription rates remain on the rise, especially for antidepressants. Insurance companies continue to reimburse only for "biologically based" conditions and cover minimal talk therapy. Pharmaceutical companies have largely unchecked power and market to both practitioners and patients alike. Consumers are influenced by these forces, as well as the broader culture of medicalization that encourages defining and solving problems through medical means. Practitioners learn their trade in this cultural and institutional context that supports the biomedical model and, in many ways, works against in-depth treatments.

Psychoanalysis beyond Psychiatry

As the biomedical model rose to dominance in psychiatry, other mental health professionals took over much of the talk therapy once provided within the field of medicine. Yet this shift was not without contention. Particularly when it came to classic psychoanalysis, American practitioners had an ongoing battle over who ought to practice psychoanalysis that began long before the rise of biomedical psychiatry. Many analysts believed that only medical doctors were trained thoroughly enough as mental health practitioners to practice psychoanalysis; prior to the 1990s, the training institutes that were affiliated with the American Psychoanalytic Association did not allow non-MDs to receive full psychoanalytic training. Though Freud was a medical doctor, he did not think highly of physicians; he reportedly called medical doctors "merchants, trading in the mitigation of miseries they scarcely attempted to understand" (Reiff 1966, 83, quoted in Conrad and Schneider 1992). Freud was an advocate of "lay analysis," or the practice of psychoanalysis by those outside the mental health fields; he did not think that medical or other professional training was a prerequisite to the practice of psychoanalysis (Conrad and Schneider 1992). Indeed, his daughter Anna Freud, the founder of child analysis, was a lay analyst. American psychoanalysts were largely at odds with Freud, whose position is best illustrated in his training of one of the most famous psychologist psychoanalysts, Theodor Reik. Though a direct descendant of Freudian psychoanalysis and one of Freud's prized students, Reik was never accepted by many American psychoanalysts because he was not an MD. From the beginning of the psychoanalytic heyday in the United States, many psychiatrists were unwilling to accept that anyone other than medical doctors was capable of practicing psychoanalysis, which, some argue, can be largely attributed to psychiatry's battle to maintain dominance over the treatment of mental illness (Abbott 1988). Because of the restrictions in the field, Reik instructed other, nonmedical practitioners interested in psychoanalysis; his lectures were the foundation for the National Psychological Association for Psychoanalysis (NPAP) in New York City, which remains an institute where many nonphysicians train in psychoanalysis.

One of the ways psychoanalysis has survived the onslaught of medicalization is that nonmedical practitioners have taken up much of the work of talk therapy. However, the opportunity to receive full training in psychoanalysis in all institutes is a relatively recent phenomenon for psychologists and social workers, who could not officially train in psychoanalysis until 1991; at this time the "Psychoanalytic Lawsuit" against the accredited institutes of the American Psychoanalytic Association was officially settled in favor of nonmedical practitioners.[13] Before then, many institutes required nonphysicians to sign a waiver promising not to practice psychoanalysis (Kalinkowitz and Aron 1998).

Though the field of psychology was highly influenced by psychodynamic theory,[14] clinical psychology training and research are also more heavily focused on short-term, evidence-based therapies and diagnosis than ever before, a function of a similar desire to be scientific, as their medically trained counterparts in psychiatry longed to be (Hunt 1993, 640). As social scientists, psychologists are not medically trained, nor are they permitted to prescribe medications.[15] The origins of psychology as a discipline are in European philosophy and behavioralism and can be traced to such figures as Immanuel Kant and Ivan Pavlov. Even if psychological practice has become much more focused on finding efficiency (e.g., cognitive behavioral therapy) for treating psychic pain than on the meaning-making process and deep explorations of the mind that characterized psychology (McWilliams 2000) and psychiatry (Hale 1995; Horwitz 2002a; Shorter 1993, 1998) for the majority of the twentieth century, it is still influenced by Freudian (and post-Freudian) theories of the mind, and some psychological training programs are still grounded in psychodynamic principles. As such, psychologists practice a significant amount of the psychodynamic psychotherapy in the United States today and may be more likely candidates to be interested in psychoanalytic theory and practice than psychiatrists. The distinction between psychodynamic psychotherapy and psychoanalysis is an important one, as the former refers simply to talking therapy that employs the basic concepts of psychodynamic theory, while the latter refers to more traditional, multiple-session-per-week treatments.

Given the relatively low enrollment in psychoanalytic training today, psychoanalytic training institutes would be in even more peril if not for the

participation of nonmedical analysts.[16] Yet in 2018, for example, at one prominent New York City psychoanalytic institute, there were six times more MDs
than non-MDs on the faculty, and eight times more candidates (trainees in the
program who had not yet graduated) were MDs, and the same was true of the
training analysts, the most powerful in the program. At another institute, seven
times more training and supervising analysts were MDs, and of the faculty overall, three times as many were MDs. Some of the most prestigious psychoanalytic training institutes still admit social workers to train only on a case-by-case
basis; debates over which practitioners are thought to be the rightful psychoanalysts still figure prominently in the field. Despite the dwindling role of psychoanalysis in psychiatry at large, psychiatrists still dominate a number of top
psychoanalytic training institutes, as exemplified by how few nonpsychiatrists
are in positions of power (or enrolled at all) in some of these programs.[17]
Though the exclusion of nonmedical candidates from psychoanalytic training
has passed, the long-standing debate still impacts the field.

The Biomedical Model Is Settled

From the 1950s into the early 1980s, psychodynamic theory was dominant in
psychiatric training, and psychoanalytic practices flourished, especially in major
U.S. cities. The last four decades in psychiatry have been characterized by the
triumph of the biomedical model; there has been a radical alteration in the theory and practice of American psychiatry in a relatively short period, which, in
many ways, represents a return to pre-Freudian theories. For a paradigm that
cannot offer the identification of a physical lesion, as with a broken bone or a
blocked artery, the biomedical model in psychiatry (with the help of pharmaceutical companies, managed care, and cultural trends that favor evidence-based
medicine) has been remarkably successful at shifting the dominant conceptualizations of mental illness—arguably as successful as Freudians were in the mid-
twentieth century at imbuing American psychiatry and American culture more
broadly with psychoanalytic ideas.

Today, the psychodynamic approach rarely exists in its ideal-typical representation with four or five meetings per week over many years. While basic
psychodynamic principles—like the notion that the relationship between the
therapist and patient is important and that patients have unconscious thoughts
and desires—still anchor many of the treatments offered in psychiatry and
other mental health fields today, questions about the efficacy and value of psychoanalysis have given way to a profession in which psychoanalysis is peripheral. Most contemporary psychiatrists have little to no training in anything
other than the biomedical model, and even psychologists are not commonly

psychodynamically oriented, as short-term treatments and biological thinking have taken over psychological training programs as well (McWilliams 2000). In a field and culture increasingly concerned with scientificity and the ability to identify the causal mechanisms for treatments of all kinds, psychoanalysis is seen, at best, as an art, at worst, as outmoded and ineffective. This is fueled by myriad forces, but the result is that both psychology and psychiatry students today are trained in professions that are not amenable to practicing psychodynamically informed kinds of therapies. McWilliams (2000, 373), a psychologist and analyst who has written extensively on the state of both fields, explains,

> My current students talk movingly about their fears that the world into which they will graduate will not allow them to practice psychotherapy in a way that makes any sense to them. . . . However dispirited my psychology students are, the situation of medical students, residents, interns, and beginning psychiatrists is even more dire. Recent figures on the cost of medical training show that the average debt of graduating medical students is now more than $75,000. In many programs debt exceeds $100,000. Who can afford the modest financial rewards of the psychoanalytic practitioner under these circumstances? . . . If one is a doctor, it seems there is no cachet in being a therapist.

Even when students want in-depth psychotherapy training, it is cost-prohibitive. And for medical doctors, choosing psychiatry as a specialty unless it's a largely psychopharmacological practice is not nearly as financially viable as other specialties in medicine. Moreover, if a practitioner is able to pay for the additional training required to practice psychoanalysis, she can still charge more for psychopharmacological treatments. And given that only the most elite insurance plans cover any form of intensive talk therapy, psychoanalysis is largely an unaffordable treatment option for most Americans. In the United States, psychoanalysis is practiced mostly in select places—typically near psychoanalytic centers in cities like New York, Chicago, Washington, and Los Angeles. Though it is difficult to accurately assess, only a small group is formally trained in psychoanalysis today. Practitioners wedded to this model struggle to maintain the psychodynamic tradition in a biomedical world.

In their attempts to keep psychodynamic treatments alive, analysts have adapted their treatments, where possible, by demonstrating efficacy. Schechter (2014, 5) argues that in the face of much lower demand, many analysts have had to scale down their psychoanalytic practices; while they "prize their self-definition as psychoanalyst," many practice only modified versions of the treatment. Analysts have also paid increased attention to evidence-based models (in the mold of clinical trials used to assess medication efficacy; Seligman 1995) that demonstrate in some cases equal reduction of symptoms as pharmacological treatments and increased quality of life, especially for patients with anxiety and depression, two of the most common diagnoses. Those who practice psychoanalysis argue that it is effective, and there is increasing evidence that shows psychotherapy may be as effective as medications for reducing symptoms and increasing quality of life for patients with some of the most common conditions like anxiety and depression (McWilliams 2000; Busch, Milrod, and Sandberg 2009; Graf, Milrod, and Aronson 2010; Leichsenring and Rabung 2008; Seligman 1995). This has done little to assuage the overwhelming sense in the field and among the public that the biomedical model offers a more valid approach to treatment. Analysts have even attempted to work within a diagnostic model, clearest in the creation of the *Psychodynamic Diagnostic Manual* (PDM; PDM Taskforce 2006). The PDM was written by prominent psychoanalysts in an attempt to bring psychodynamic language and principles back into diagnosis, to educate practitioners who are coming of age in an era when the DSM is all they know, and to show that there are alternative frameworks for looking at symptoms. The PDM is introduced with the following:

> The goal of the PDM is to complement the DSM and ICD efforts of the past 30 years by explicating the broad range of mental functioning. . . . Mental health comprises more than simply the absence of symptoms. It involves a person's overall mental functioning including relationships; emotional depth, range and regulation; coping capacities; and self-observing abilities. Just as healthy cardiac functioning cannot be defined simply as an absence of chest pain, healthy mental functioning is more than the absence of observable symptoms of psychopathology. It involves the full range of human cognitive, emotional and behavioral capacities. . . . That a comprehensive conceptualization of health is the foundation for describing disorder may seem self-evident, yet the mental health field has not developed its diagnostic procedures accordingly. In the last two decades, there has been an increasing tendency to define mental problems primarily on the basis of observable symptoms, behavior, and traits, with overall personality functioning and levels of adaptation noted only secondarily. (PDM Taskforce 2006, 13)[18]

Describing itself as a "complement" to the diagnostic guidelines in use in both American and global psychiatry, the PDM is ostensibly an attempt to integrate dynamic principles into mainstream mental health practice, but it represents the struggle of psychoanalysis to survive and remain relevant in a biomedical world. The PDM is not now nor is it likely to ever be used widely. In fact, the field is moving increasingly toward even more biological thinking, as is evidenced by the emergence of the National Institute of Mental Health's Research Domain Criteria (RDoC), which Whooley (2010) describes as a "brain-centric conceptualization of mental disorders." Practitioners of in-depth talk therapy are working beneath and sometimes against an immense biomedical tide. Furthermore, some argue that the very model of randomized controlled trials is inapplicable to most forms of talk therapy, especially psychoanalysis, and even CBT given the low external validity and reliability of a number of studies of this type (Fonagy 2003).

Given this history, I now turn to my interviewees' ideas about their field, their patients, and their profession. Their narratives offer insight into how the biomedical model retains its central role in the field as well as how psychodynamic principles have managed to survive the biomedical revolution, albeit in a much less central role for most practitioners. In the narratives of the psychiatrists and psychologists I spoke with are clues to many of the key issues in practice today, how they stem from those that have long been present in the field, but also how practitioners use these seemingly dichotomous models in practice.

Chapter 2

Practitioner Portraits and Pathways to Practice

In this chapter I offer an in-depth look at four of the forty-three practitioners I spoke with. These narratives provide insight into how different kinds of practitioners think about their work and their field more broadly. These portraits are the point of departure for the key issues that structure the chapters to follow— namely, how interviewees feel about and use the treatment tools available to them by virtue of their psychiatry, psychology, or psychoanalytic training, and what it's like to treat patients in their respective fields.

From here on out, I refer to the psychiatrists I spoke with who are not psychoanalysts as "Biomedical Psychiatrists," as their primary mode of treatment is the biomedical model, by which I mean diagnosis and psychopharmacology. I dub psychiatrists who are also psychoanalysts "Biodynamic Psychiatrists" because they are trained in multiple paradigms: the biomedical and the psychodynamic. And finally, I refer to the psychologists trained as analysts as "Psychodynamic Psychologists," as they were largely trained in in-depth talk therapy of the psychodynamic tradition in graduate school and then as specialists in psychoanalytic practice and theory.[1] Despite these ideal typical categorizations, each doctor has unique elements of her pathway to practice and personal reasons for being drawn to the mental health profession. Yet the kinds of stories these doctors tell—of parents who are mental health practitioners, of influential childhood figures, of a propensity for thinking about the mind, or of a decision about what kind of practice they wanted to have—*are* characteristic of others in their group. The descriptions of training, at least in basic structure, are identical for all practitioners in each of the three groups.

I offer portraits of two separate Biomedical Psychiatrists as there was a divide between those whose practices were almost entirely biomedical (psychopharmacologists) and those who had at least a handful of patients in talk therapy. The Biodynamic Psychiatrists' practices also varied by their age and psychiatry training cohort, but their general attitudes toward the field and descriptions of their patients were more similar, as was the case for the Psychodynamic Psychologists. The portraits provide insight into the way a doctor in each of these groups might be inclined to respond to the variety of topics addressed in my conversations with them, and insights into the way in which the biomedical and psychodynamic paradigms impact their thinking and practice.

Dr. Evans, MD: Biomedical Psychiatrist

Dr. Evans practices in a pristine office building in Downtown Manhattan; it is sparkling clean, sterile—hospital-like. An administrative assistant for what I surmised was likely a dozen doctors in the complex greeted me from her desk as I walked through the front entrance. Dr. Evans was one of only three doctors I interviewed who had a staff and practiced in a setting reminiscent of other fields of medicine; most psychiatrists and psychologists in private practice in New York City have offices in suites that they share with one or two other practitioners, along with shared waiting rooms and bathrooms. The sheer cost of an office staff indicated to me that Dr. Evans must see a significant number of patients per day, as did the difficulty in scheduling an appointment with her. I was originally scheduled to interview Dr. Evans in 2008, but her secretary called me on several occasions to postpone, and finally could not find another time for her to see me. I moved on to other interviewees, hoping to come back to her at the end of the interviewing process, which is how I finally wound up in her office in 2011 after at least a few weeks of phone tag and schedule manipulations. Dr. Evans could offer me only forty minutes, which turned into about thirty because she was running behind schedule when I arrived; there was already a patient waiting for her while we talked. It turned out that thirty minutes was more than enough time, as Dr. Evans's practice did not lend itself to many of the questions I asked of the psychoanalysts in the study; Dr. Evans does not practice talk therapy at all and had little to say about the matter. The short length of this portrait is reflective of the brevity of our conversation.

Though both of us were aware of the looming time constraints, Dr. Evans was welcoming and attentive. In her early fifties, she was an energetic conversationalist and had a youthful quality, which I recall thinking made sense for someone whose patients are largely children and young adults. Our interview began as most did, with a discussion of her decision to become a psychiatrist and the pathway she took to practicing psychiatry. Dr. Evans considers herself a psychopharmacologist; her business card is inscribed accordingly, signifying a practice that revolves largely around the prescribing of psychotropic medications. Of her approximately five hundred patients, Dr. Evans sees five for what she calls "talk therapy." Though she describes these patients as her "regulars," she sees them a few times a month or less, and her version of talk therapy largely revolves around discussions of medication side effects and basic life events.

Dr. Evans enjoys practicing psychopharmacology, although one of the primary reasons she became a psychiatrist was because of her interest in a medical field that was about more than the mechanics of the body; she wanted to be in a profession that would allow her to have a real relationship with her patients. When I asked her why she decided to become a psychiatrist, she told me,

> So, I was starting out to be a pediatrician and then in medical school I actually spent two summers doing surgery because I thought I was gonna be a surgeon. I didn't quite like the fact that in surgery you don't get the chance to really speak to the patient. And then I think probably for me, when I was doing my clinical rotations in my third year and pediatric was like my first one. My second one was psychiatry and I kinda like—I thought those were the two greatest things I had done, and I just sorta merged the two and then just kinda continued with it . . . I got sorta turned on by it.

Dr. Evans valued her experiences practicing medicine of the body, but a desire to know more about patients and have a more meaningful interchange with them drew her to psychiatry. And so she followed her four years of medical school, which is characterized by studies of bodily functioning, with four years of a psychiatry residency, where she learned to diagnose and prescribe appropriate medications in a hospital setting. The first year of residency is an internship, the first half of which is hands-on medical training. It is the only hands-on medical experience involved in becoming a psychiatrist. The second half of the internship year is the beginning of work in an inpatient setting, which involves treating psychiatric patients in a hospital setting using medications and talk therapy. Talk therapy is not always part of the training today and was not for Dr. Evans. Psychiatry residents spend much of their time prescribing medication. In a hospital setting, a team of people is responsible for each patient; psychologists and social workers are much more likely to be the providers of talk therapy. Part of the way in which psychiatrists become so adept at diagnosing and prescribing is because that is generally their main (if not only) role in hospital settings.

The last three years of psychiatry training, known as psychiatry residency proper, involve a combination of treatment in inpatient hospital settings and outpatient settings, where patients come to the hospital for a session and then return home. In addition, Dr. Evans and all psychiatrists are required to do rounds in the hospital, and attend case conferences, where individual cases are presented to an audience of residents as a training exercise. In the last two years, residents undergo one-on-one supervision of their cases, intensive class work in diagnostics, the brain, and medications, and a small amount of course work in talk therapy. Finally, Dr. Evans completed an additional two years of a fellowship in child psychiatry, which is required in order to work with children.

Dr. Evans attended medical school and finished her residency years in the 1980s, during the height of the radical changes in psychiatry. When I asked her about the shift from the psychodynamic model to the biomedical model in psychiatry training and practice, she told me there are "definitely more positives." She elaborated, "We have a better understanding of the brain, the nervous system, mechanism of action, of medications, and I think the real biology behind something that's still stigmatized in a lot of areas. So I see actually much more positives. I'm not sure what I would say are the negatives." Dr. Evans did not point to anything problematic or lacking in the medical model or biomedical treatment. For her, the availability of new medicines and the centrality of the biomedical model in psychiatry have led only to advancements. While Dr. Evans thinks the DSM is useful for clinicians, and she indicated its centrality to her practice, she did offer one critique of the DSM when I asked about it directly:

> The problem is if you stay too structured you may not kind of open up things more to see—I guess in some ways you don't want to over diagnose. . . . And I think you don't want to kinda box yourself in. Like the power of suggestion. I think it's good to use as a blueprint or a structure but not everybody's gonna fit it. Especially with kids because I think the DSM was really mostly made for adults. They really don't fit into their boxes. They're still in kinda a state of development.

The DSM, she explained, promotes the idea that people "fit into their boxes," which she indicates can impact the way clinicians think about their patients beyond the symptoms presented in an initial assessment and can be particularly problematic for children, who are still developing. Overall, however, she described the DSM as "very comprehensive" and explained the importance of its exhaustiveness: "It's very structured, so I think in that sense it's very beneficial because you go through—it's very comprehensive. I think you go through current symptoms, but you also ask just kinda lifetime things. And I think if you fall back on a structured thing that's based on DSM, you're not going to omit anything. Is really kind of all-inclusive." Upon meeting new patients, Dr. Evans engages in what she describes as a thorough diagnostic interview. Illustrating her process in terms of her child patients, since they make up the majority of her practice, Dr. Evans explains the important factors needed to diagnose: "I need historical perspective. I need teacher reports, any testing. I usually ask if they've had psych testing. I talk to the teachers. I talk to other people in the lives of the child. I really sit down with the parents and get kind of an elaborate chronological order of symptoms as kind of a gold standard. And then a very thorough history, including a family history." Dr. Evans uses checklists geared toward diagnosis of psychiatric symptoms that are based on DSM categories, so even when she doesn't consult the DSM directly, its categories are still highly influential in her diagnosis. It is not only symptoms that Dr. Evans assesses, particularly when diagnosing children, as she describes above when she details the range of considerations including important adults in the child's life and school performance. Yet when I asked her what the etiology of psychiatric conditions is, she replied simply, "Genetics. Genetics. Genetics." After a few moments' pause she added, "and environment," but made sure to clarify, "the genetics will predispose to a particular response," even when there is a clear environmental stimulus.

Perhaps most indicative of the nature of Dr. Evans's psychiatric practice was her response when I asked what role she thinks medication plays in treatment. She looked at me, confused, as if pleading for an explanation as she said, "What do you mean *the role*?" I began to explain, but got only two words out when she interrupted me to add, "I think it is treatment. Especially for something like ADHD or depression or anxiety." For the disorders for which she sees a clear diagnosis, and for which medicines are considered effective and relatively benign, medication is *the* treatment. She was careful to add that many of her patients are in talk therapy with another therapist; she was unclear about why exactly she felt it was important to make sure to enforce the idea that her patients are in combined treatments, although my guess is because it's the gold standard in the field. But for her, medication is treatment. Also indicative of how Dr. Evans thinks about her field are her thoughts about the contribution psychiatry makes to society. She told me, "I think our field has grown tremendously in neuroscience and biology. I think it's really destigmatizing mental illness. I think it's really getting us far greater understanding of etiology and hopefully the early identification and treatment." For her, the goal of psychiatry is to continue to advance biomedical treatments and, she hopes, for technology to aid in identifying underlying biological markers of illness.

Dr. Sutter, MD: Biomedical Psychiatrist

Dr. Sutter's office is in an affluent suburb of New York City, where beautiful tall trees line the streets and the air is heavy with the smell of freshly cut grass. On an April afternoon she greeted me in the waiting room of her suburban office building, as she was still in mid-conversation with someone via a Bluetooth headset. For a few moments, I could not tell if she was talking to the person on the phone or me. Dr. Sutter was apologetic about the delay, yet we would be interrupted several times during our conversation by her incoming calls and texts, even though this was clearly not a work day for her; she was dressed informally and referred to having come from dropping her kids off somewhere nearby. Though she was kind and helpful, she had obviously fit me into a solidly booked day of nonprofessional activity, and there was, therefore, a sense of urgency about finishing in the allotted time. This, however, did not present a problem as we completed the interview, even with some pauses for unanticipated phone conversation, within forty minutes. Though Dr. Sutter was not as pithy as Dr. Evans, we had plenty of time, which was the case with most of the Biomedical Psychiatrists.

Dr. Sutter was born in the late 1950s and grew up in the New York City area. She attended an Ivy League school and began medical school in the early 1980s. She therefore moved into her internship and residency at the outset of the biomedical heyday and did so at a top hospital in New York City. At the time of our meeting, Dr. Sutter had about seventy-five patients in her practice, about fifteen of whom she saw on a regular basis, which for her is generally once a week. The remaining sixty of her patients saw her either for brief behavioral therapy (e.g., CBT) or sporadic medication management. Her practice was much smaller than Dr. Evans's, in part because she starts most of her patients in combined treatments (talk therapy and medication).

> I have a lot of people where I start them with combined. I have very few people who I just do therapy with. I think most people don't go to a psychiatrist anymore if they don't need meds. I have a lot of people I'll start with in combined therapy and meds seeing once a week, or some of those that I'll see twice a week and then go to once a week. So, the therapy needs will wane and I'll see them just for meds then. I'd say that's a lot of my med patients, although I do take some patients just for meds.

Many of the patients Dr. Sutter starts out seeing for therapy ultimately become very infrequent mediation patients or do not come for therapy at all after a certain point, which she attributes to the state of the field—namely that the primary work of psychiatry is psychopharmacology. When I asked her if she has any patients who are not on medications, she told me she "started this little niche of couples and family treatment." "Right now," she told me, "I'm seeing two regular hours of that. I'm not medicating any of those people. I have one patient who I'm not medicating, I guess, and I'm seeing her for therapy. But I will medicate her. I'm just trying to figure out what she needs. She needs something." Aside from an anomaly of two families, who come to counseling for specific relationship problems rather than for psychiatric symptoms, Dr. Sutter's practice is dominated by psychopharmacological treatment, and when she uses talk therapy, it is for practical, nondiagnosable problems.

As was typical, we began our conversation by discussing why Dr. Sutter decided to become a psychiatrist, which she describes having considered even before medical school: "I went to medical school thinking that I might be a psychiatrist, either that or family practice. My father was a psychiatrist and my mother was an internist so I sort of had, like I knew about both. I was pretty sure I wanted to do psychiatry. I had done some crisis intervention stuff; I worked at a shelter for battered women and I'd done lots of stuff like that before. But it was really during the third year that I decided definitely I was more interested in the psychiatry part." Given that she did not definitively choose psychiatry as her specialty until her third year of medical school, I asked her if there was something about the field that set it apart from other branches of medicine, or what it was that really drew her to psychiatry rather than another medical specialty. She explained that she thinks it was "a combination of interest in having long-term relationships with patients in a pretty intimate kind of way that you don't really get in the rest of medicine. . . . And just feeling like I could really make a difference in people's lives." Though Dr. Sutter had a clearer idea that she would specialize in psychiatry than did Dr. Evans, she too chose psychiatry over other medical specialties for the potential relationships with patients.

Our conversation then turned to the major changes Dr. Sutter has seen in psychiatry since she trained in the 1980s.

I mean, the huge thing that happened is that medicine changed since I trained. Managed care hit when I was a resident. . . . [Before, insurance] paid like ninety percent of therapy for residents like once or twice a week for the whole year. It was endless, endless coverage. There's not that kind of coverage anymore for residents or anyone. Insurance coverage changed and it just drove huge changes. I'd say fifty to seventy-five percent of my prescriptions that I write for patients, I have to call the insurance company to get a preauthorization. It's a total waste of time because they always approve it, or they usually approve it. I don't know why. It's just a waste of time. I used to be able to write a prescription and that didn't used to happen, so there's all this managing. . . . What is good is that first of all, almost all of the medications that we use now weren't around when I was training. They're all new and they're all better. There's much more choice and effective medications, which is probably why you can do really effective psychopharmacology now in the way that you were just beginning to then . . . things have so many less side effects and there's so much more array of choices of what you could use.

Dr. Sutter expressed a sense of progress in psychiatry, which she associated specifically with the newest medications, even though she was forthright about her distaste for the proscription of treatment by insurance companies. Likewise, she told me, forces beyond her control impact the kind of treatment she provides:

There have certainly been people who come in here for evaluations where I'll say to them that I don't think they need medication or that the medication that they need is so uncomplicated that they could see a psychiatrist infrequently and save some money by going to a non-MD for therapy. I certainly do say that to people. . . . I think the economy changed things a lot, and insurance changed things a lot, so that people who are willing to pay for a psychiatrist have enough money that they don't care. There are people who think you should only go to a psychiatrist for treatment because they'll be better than other people. No matter what you'd say, which I don't necessarily believe. I mean, one of my office mates is a nurse practitioner. I'm her supervising psychiatrist. She's worked at [a hospital in New York] forever. You can't do better than going to her. There are people who would never go to a nurse practitioner. So, there's plenty of sort of bread-and-butter depression, anxiety that I treat for whatever reasons.

Given her clientele, which is largely upper-middle class, Dr. Sutter's treatments are not often heavily swayed by outside forces, but it is certainly the case that a patient looking for talk therapy alone may seek out a psychologist, social worker, nurse practitioner, or other kind of counselor to save money. This inevitably impacts the type of treatment Dr. Sutter most often provides; before she ever meets a patient, those seeking talk therapy may self-select out of seeing a psychiatrist and opt to see a practitioner who charges less per session for talk therapy.

For a range of reasons, prescribing medication is a primary part of Dr. Sutter's practice. When I asked her what indicates that someone should be on medication, she explained, "You know, I think certainly if they have mental illness that responds to medications. So, sometimes it's one hundred percent clear that someone needs medication because they have a clear-cut depression." For some patients, Dr. Sutter feels certain medications are indicated, but she also explains that she divides her patients into three categories when they come into her office:

> I think of the people who, they just need medication. There's no question. And I'll say to them, "I think it would really be a huge mistake for you not to try a medication." Those are the people where they have serious depression or serious anxiety or serious attention deficit disorder or some bipolar disorder or psychosis—things that medications work really well for. It's just stupid not to take them. So, it's like having high blood pressure. You wouldn't go into a doctor's office and say, "I'm gonna talk to you about your high blood pressure and try and help mellow you out." You'd say, "Look, you have blood pressure that could really kill you and it's making your life—it's gonna cause all sorts of bad things, so you need medicine." Those people I say, "I really think it would be a huge mistake if you don't take medicine." Then there's the group of people where I say it's sort of optional, where I think it would help, but they could decide and they have to weigh the pros and cons and the side effects. It's not that medicines are side effect free. And I'll discuss the side effects with them and then I'll say to them, "You know, you can try and you'll decide if you think it's helping or not." . . . Those are the people who have sort of mild depression or mild anxiety where cognitive behavioral therapy or some sort of therapy can make a big difference in terms of learning various relaxation techniques . . . someone who has panic attacks, someone who has phobia of planes, for instance, you can give them medicine. But also, my office mate . . . does amazing cognitive behavioral therapy with anxiety disorders. I say to them, "There's a treatment. It works really well. It's not drugs. You will get cured and you could do that."

In drawing a parallel to high blood pressure, Dr. Sutter is clear about her doctorly roll in treating her more severely ill patients. But there are also patients who have less severe symptoms and for whom she still believes medications are helpful, though with them she feels less obligated to push for medications. This thinking is rooted in the DSM model, which assesses severity and duration. For instance, the patient who is phobic of planes has an acute symptom with a clear stimulus. The patient could take a medicine as needed when at high altitudes, for example, or could try to work it out in a problem-focused therapy like CBT. On the other hand, the patient who has many panic attacks over the course of a day with no clear-cut stimulus and cannot focus on work or school would be a much more likely candidate for Dr. Sutter to strongly recommend medication. Dr. Sutter also describes a third group of people who do not need or who cannot take medication: "I just think they don't need medicine. Or they can't be on the medicines. I have one guy who had a heart attack and he really needs medicine for ADHD but he can't be on it. Or I have another guy who had a congenital heart problem and again, he really needed ADHD medicine. . . . You teach them the technique, I mean, there are lots of things that people who have ADHD can do to help themselves organize themselves that they do anyway when they're on medicine." Dr. Sutter lumps patients who do not need medications and those who cannot take them into one category in part because her role is the same—she has to find a nonmedicinal alternative. This third group is the least relevant to her practice; again, for a range of reasons, patients who do not need medicines are less likely to end up in a psychiatrist's office these days. She seems to lament, for a brief moment, that today, if patients do not need medicine, they do not necessarily need to see a psychiatrist, a quite different response from Dr. Evans.

The centrality of psychopharmacology in her practice maps onto Dr. Sutter's thinking about the etiology of mental illness, which she says has "two components": "I think that if you look at study after study it's usually borne out . . . it's the biology and the environment and it's the interplay of the two of those. And the biological component is huge, but then the environment is also huge. And when I say biology I'm speaking very broadly; not just genetics, but environmental—all the crap that our bodies have been exposed to and trauma and you know pregnancy and whatever." While she mentions trauma and environmental factors, it is in passing rather than as a central influence on etiology; her focus is on biological factors, and the environment is described in terms of toxins and prenatal exposure. This mentality fits with the use of medications— if biology underlies all experiences, including environmental influences, it is therefore logical that medicines can help even conditions that do not stem from genetic causes.

When I asked her what role the DSM plays in her practice, Dr. Sutter responded, as most of my interviewees did, by saying, "very little," and she laughed in a manner that insinuated she thinks little of the manual's utility. However, she continued,

> It plays a few different roles. One is that you have to put a diagnosis down for insurance, and I try and have that diagnosis be accurate . . . partly because it becomes record. I don't wanna commit fraud. I don't wanna label people with things they don't have because that's a bad thing. . . . So with someone who's depressed, I would wanna be thinking, "Is this just a standard depression or is this someone who has some sort of bipolar disorder going on," because that would definitely mean I would think differently in terms of the medication treatment. But I'm very careful about labeling. For people who wanna know their diagnoses, I'm always saying, "It's like seeing your brown hair. It doesn't say that much about it." I'm not a labeling person . . . I don't think my practice is un-DSM-related. I think about it and I have one on my desk and I pull it out regularly to look at and put numbers down and stuff, but it's just a little too simplistic.

The importance of careful diagnosis, for Dr. Sutter, is largely to avoid unnecessary or problematic labeling, which makes sense given that she believes the contribution psychiatry has made to society is largely to do with destigmatizing mental illness. She says she has, over her career, "seen mental illness go from being really stigmatized and really hidden and too many people not getting help for what their problems are to it being much more acceptable to get help and to the help that we have being much more effective." She feels strongly in terms of "both medication and therapy, we have just so many more, way more effective treatments than they had twenty-five years ago." Dr. Sutter believes in the significant advances of her field, which she attributes to routinized treatments like CBT and to new medications.

I wanted to know how Dr. Sutter, as a clinician who relies on accurate diagnosis, feels about the DSM and how she uses it in her practice. When I asked her if she could think about any issues with the DSM, she responded, "Just that it's sort of cookbooky and doesn't tell you that much about a person." But when I asked her what the greatest strengths of the DSM are, she responded exactly the same way: "That it's cookbooky." She explained further that because of the DSM "everyone knows what major depression means and that when you read a study and it says, 'The people in the study were diagnosed with major depression recurrent, you know who they are.' When it says, 'They didn't have substance abuse or they didn't have borderline personality,' you just know who those people are and then you could sort of think of your own patients." The

DSM makes it possible for practitioners to communicate with one another, to understand the studies they read, and to make associations between those studies and what is going on with their own patients. It provides them with a shared language with which to discuss illnesses and patients. Even though this allows practitioners to do their job, it is also limiting—for Dr. Sutter, the strengths and weaknesses of the diagnostic model are one and the same.

When I asked Dr. Sutter more specifically about the role of medication in treatment, she told me, "I think it's a really important modality of treatment that could really make a huge difference. Sometimes it completely gets rid of symptoms really quickly or not quickly enough, but it really can change people's lives." Unlike Dr. Evans, her more psychopharmacologically oriented counterpart, Dr. Sutter describes medication not as treatment, but rather as one part of it. One central purpose of her talk therapy sessions is for discussing experiences with medications:

> I don't know if you call that therapy, but there's being a doctor, sort of discussing the medication and talking about the pros and cons of it and why you take it and why it's important to take as prescribed. Or if you're not gonna take it as prescribed, call me and tell me about it. You don't like it, don't wanna take it again, let's figure out what you're gonna do. I spend a lot of time talking about that stuff with meds. But then, most of the people coming to see me have big, for instance, lived a year where you've gotten breast cancer and had your husband maybe leave and your mother die, the medicine's not gonna fix all that. So there was a lot of talk that needed to be done. . . . Most of the people that walk in my office have some of them huge life issues going on.

She is clear that medicine won't fix everything and that she spends time talking to patients about their lives, but she is also clear that a major part of talk therapy, for her, involves discussing the effects of the medications she has prescribed. Dr. Sutter did not seem to associate the term "talk therapy" with psychodynamic psychotherapy.

Dr. Nelson, MD: Biodynamic Psychiatrist

Dr. Nelson and I met at her office on the Upper West Side of Manhattan on a warm June afternoon. Though she was only the fifth practitioner I interviewed, I had already become accustomed to the routine interchanges with doormen, who are often skeptical of unknown faces, but always acquiesce at the mention of "Dr. so and so"; practitioners generally inform the guardians of their buildings not to ask for any identifying information to protect patients' confidentiality.

And so I was granted entry and made my way to a small but ornate elevator that would deposit me at the familiar low-lit, narrow halls customary to prewar buildings.

Dr. Nelson was right on time, and as we talked, she struck me as direct and concise, but equally thoughtful. Our interview finished in a little under the scheduled forty-five minutes, which was unusual for the analysts, who tended to go over our allotted time, often because they asked about my work and my training and responded to questions with extensive description. Because we had a few minutes to spare at the end of the interview, we had a chance to talk a little more informally, during which time Dr. Nelson suggested the brevity might have been because she needed less time to mull over my questions since she teaches at her psychoanalytic institute and has an academic interest in many of the topics we discussed. I could tell she thinks extensively about her treatment approach and about etiology. After all, she spends a great deal of time discussing these very issues with her students. She spoke with ease about many of the key issues some of her colleagues needed time to sort through. This, however, also increased my need to draw her out, as her sometimes-incorrect assumption seemed to be that her answers were self-explanatory or that she and I had the same knowledge base.

Dr. Nelson was born at the close of the 1950s and was raised in and around New York City. She attended a series of elite schools in the Northeast and started four years of medical school at the tail end of the 1970s. Dr. Nelson describes what she calls "the development of her interest in psychiatry" as something that emerged during medical school.

When I went to medical school, I thought I was going to do some kind of community health, public health. I was somewhat of an activist before I went to medical school and I worked doing organizing, and just eventually decided that I wanted more technical skills to offer people. And so medical school just seemed like the most humanistic approach to getting technical skills. I was doing environmental work and instead of continuing. . . . I shifted towards health care, but then in medical school it really just took me by surprise how much I liked psychiatry, and rather than train as a physician, as an internist or a surgeon or a dermatologist, and then yet still figure out a way how to apply it and integrate it with my politics, I just sort of went the other direction and decided that I was most interested intellectually in psychiatry and why not just do it? . . . I just really like being with patients and thinking about, observing how their minds worked and relating to them in therapy. And emotionally I just thought the whole mind, body thing was fascinating, so I just sort of went with my gut on what was intellectually interesting to me.

Like that of her Biomedical Psychiatrist counterparts, Drs. Evans and Sutter, Dr. Nelson's drive toward psychiatry grew from its differences from other medical specialties; psychiatry allowed for more communication with patients and more time with them. In addition, Dr. Nelson described her decision to be a psychiatrist as a way to make a contribution to humanity and to pursue intellectually interesting questions through her work—her practice is a direct way to retain what she sees as a "humanistic approach," by which I took her to mean person-centered or patient-centered. She also considered her personal life when choosing psychiatry and particularly private practice, as it allows practitioners to control their schedule and integrate time for family and career, unlike, for instance, in surgery or obstetrics, where the timing of procedures is often unpredictable. She began training when there was still a significant presence of talk therapy (specifically psychodynamic psychotherapy) training in residency programs, though even then, just before the release of DSM-III, the focus was shifting toward diagnosis and prescribing practices and had certainly crystallized as such by the time she graduated.

Dr. Nelson practiced for approximately six years and then entered five years of psychoanalytic training in the late 1980s. As is the case for all psychoanalysts, Dr. Nelson was in treatment with a training analyst (who has vast experience in the field and has been through a rigorous certification process), which is a mandatory part of the requirement to become a certified psychoanalyst. This meant paying for treatment four times per week and losing the same number of hours when she could see her own patients. Dr. Nelson also had to take on three analytic cases (four sessions per week per case) over the course of the five years. Each of these cases had to be supervised by a different training analyst, which amounts to an additional forty-five minutes per case per week. These sessions are generally at a reduced fee since practitioners are in training, which means giving up additional income. Finally, all five years of training include course work. At the same time trainees perform their routine duties—for instance, seeing their regular patients and teaching psychiatry residents. Given that the training in psychoanalysis is cumbersome and costly, I asked Dr. Nelson why she decided to pursue it. She explained,

> In psychiatry residency, we had lots of different teachers and the teachers who I found most engaging intellectually, and who I also developed the most rapport with were the analysts . . . I was gravitating towards them as mentors. And then I really liked working one on one with patients

and eventually . . . I was trying to integrate having a family, and being somewhat available and balance work and family life. I was toying with how to do it all, how to at least find whatever it is that I had to work at intellectually interesting that I started feeling like private practice was probably most likely going to be the emphasis. And I was interested in psychoanalysis and developing my therapy skills and working further with those mentors from the analytic institute, and so it came together really as a decision as a way to integrate work and family.

The training in residency to prepare a psychiatrist to practice in-depth talk therapy was minimal at best, which left a void for Dr. Nelson, who wanted to be a good talk therapist. She felt she was not ready after psychiatry training alone to have the kind of practice that would be fulfilling to her unless she trained as an analyst.

At the time of her interview, Dr. Nelson had approximately fifty patients in her practice. Though she is a psychoanalyst, she sees about twenty patients infrequently for medication only. She has five patients who are in analysis, which means she sees them four times a week, for forty-five minutes each session. Therefore, a considerable number of her patient hours—in fact, about twenty hours per week (an "hour" is forty five minutes)—are spent practicing psychoanalysis. This is more than is typical of most analysts today. Fifteen of Dr. Nelson's patients do not take any medications, which means about one-third of her practice is strictly talk therapy treatment. She sees some patients twice per week for in-depth, psychodynamic psychotherapy, a common treatment frequency for Biomedical Psychiatrists who aim to use their psychoanalytic perspective in treatment, even if they cannot (because of financial or other reasons) see many of their patients in a traditional, four-session analysis.

Dr. Nelson explains that the most important contribution psychiatry has made to society is that it provides a particular kind of health care that "takes care of people's emotional well-being and treats their mental illnesses." She describes psychiatry as an essential component of the medical system. Pausing for pointed laughter as she hit terms such as "evidence-based" and jokes about her colleagues taking the psychotropic medicines they prescribe, Dr. Nelson summarized her thoughts about the dominant treatment modality in psychiatry today: "In mainstream American psychiatry I would say it's medical model, DSM-based, where people make diagnoses and then offer treatments based on the diagnoses, some of which are evidence-based. But I think the dominant thrust right now is in medications for psychiatrists—I mean for psychiatrists to prescribe, and take if they wish. And I think talking therapies have been less popular, but there are a group of them that are evidence-based that still remain cornerstone in mainstream psychiatry."[2] She indicated an awareness of being part of a small, local group of therapists, and she wanted me to know that psychiatrists in other parts of the country would likely be less oriented toward talk therapy and much more toward biomedical treatments. She also noted that this is in part because of the availability in New York City of patients who can afford to pay for treatment that is not reimbursed by insurance companies, whereas in most other parts of the country (even elsewhere in New York State), patients are more limited by what treatment their insurance company will pay for. Patients with fewer resources and in other parts of the country are also less likely to know non-biomedical treatments are available since it's unlikely they will encounter a practitioner trained in any form of psychodynamic psychotherapy. Practitioners are keenly aware of how these structural and cultural factors impact them at the local level and shape psychiatric practice more generally.

Because she considers herself part of a minority that practices psychoanalysis, Dr. Nelson is sensitive to differences between psychoanalysis and the biomedical treatments psychiatrists so commonly offer. She explains which patients are likely to engage in and benefit from psychoanalysis:

> In terms of psychoanalysis in my practice, I see it as the way to offer the deepest treatment experience. And it fits a niche in terms of treating people who are suffering from sort of coping problems and character problems. The group of people who would take advantage of it are often people who would take advantage of other modalities, so they may also use medications and other kinds of therapies before entering psychoanalysis, but the psychoanalysis offers the most intensive, rigorous approach to personality and character problems and higher-level neurotic problems for those who have the motivation to do it.

In her description of psychoanalytic treatment, Dr. Nelson took a pragmatic approach. She explained that people with neurotic problems as well as those who are motivated to understand themselves benefit the most from it. She was also sure to mention that in-depth talk therapy is usefully combined with medication treatment, a common notion for most practitioners today.

When it comes to her professional identity, Dr. Nelson finds her role as a Biodynamic Psychiatrist complicated. She describes the difficulties of maintaining full membership in two different professional communities: the psychoanalytic and mainstream, biomedical psychiatric. Becoming a psychoanalyst did not come naturally for Dr. Nelson, as someone who was drawn to medical training, even though she was interested in it and felt motivated to become an adept talk therapist. However, about a decade after her analytic training, she now feels much more aligned with other analysts than she does with mainstream, Biomedical Psychiatrists. She describes the experience of being both a psychoanalyst and a psychiatrist:

> I really see myself more and more sub-specializing in psychoanalysis and psychoanalytic therapies, so that's probably what I'm best at. And I've had to tolerate that I'm not best at general psychiatry, but that I'm a good enough pharmacologist for what most people need. And then I use consultations when I get out of my range and so that's really been the transition: the sort of accepting that I may be expert at one thing, but not at something else. . . . For me, really learning how to get good at psychoanalysis has taken a huge amount of work and it would be hard for me to also put the work into keeping up with the cutting edge of pharmacology at the same time.

Dr. Nelson takes the question of how it feels to be both an analyst and a psychiatrist quite literally when she describes her lack of ability to be expert at both. Her description was of an almost painstaking decision to give up being a really good psychopharmacologist in order to be a better psychoanalyst. The difficulty is in part because psychiatric training is so greatly about being a good medical doctor and using the tools of the biomedical model. However, Dr. Nelson voiced little difficulty in practicing using both paradigms for the majority of patients. She manages the medications for the average patient and sends the more complicated cases to a psychopharmacologist. Though she has had to make some concessions in her own identity as a psychiatrist, the problems she has faced have mostly been in trying to stay equally adept at and informed about the latest treatments in both paradigms.

Dr. Nelson and I discussed the role medication plays in psychiatric treatment. She explained that it is "the shortest route to alleviate pain." She told me, "If someone fits into a DSM diagnosis that medicine treats, I basically feel like it's my obligation as a physician to offer it up," though she added that it won't necessarily alleviate complex forms of suffering. She described pain as something acute (a specific symptom for instance) and suffering as more of an ongoing experience that extends beyond symptomatology (the consequence of pain). She also alluded to the biomedical model as more apt to tackle the former, while the psychodynamic has the potential to dig deeper and potentially address suffering.

As is also typical of Biodynamic Practitioners, Dr. Nelson clearly identifies herself as a medical doctor; she sees diagnosis and the efficient treatment of pain as essential parts of her job. In doing so, an initial diagnosis is important, even if there is much more to a treatment:

> I know in the back of my mind that I'm gonna write some kind of diagnosis, but I don't feel like I necessarily have to know what it is after one meeting, so mostly I'm trying to get the story and figure out what's going on and what does the person need. If a diagnosis easily pops up the first time, I will put it in the chart. . . . I mean I take a good history and I take a family history. I review a list of symptoms to see if they do fit together in a diagnosis. You know a medical history and drugs, substances all. I do a medical as well as a psychiatric evaluation.

Though she does not use a standard checklist, when she refers to diagnosis, Dr. Nelson means thinking of the DSM symptoms a patient has. On the role of the DSM in her practice, she says,

> I think it is important to label what we see both because of using medications and in terms of picking therapies, as therapies start to get tested for certain diagnoses. But the fine-tuning of, you know, whether someone has one form of anxiety or another—I don't usually bother with very much . . . I really see it as a tool to help us talk to each other and label what we see. . . . My goal is not to try to use it . . . it probably is a good thing to continue to develop but it's just not something I'm interested in focusing on. I mean I'm glad it's there and I think it's a good endeavor and should be continued and that over time it will better approximate, I hope, what in fact these syndromes are.

She takes a distant approach to DSM, making sure to note that she really has little interest in it at all. As she described the role of the DSM, she chuckled, as if indicating the useless, silly nature of the manual, but she was also careful to point out that while the DSM is not very useful and plays only a peripheral role in her practice, the biomedical model itself is central. Seeing the ironic nature of her own critique of the DSM and simultaneously strong adherence to the biomedical model, she laughed again, as she said, "The categories [in DSM] and like the long lists don't feel like the way I'd approach it so much, but I think it is a medical model tool and probably not that far off from what I said I do use." Dr. Nelson comes full circle from saying DSM has little role to acknowledging that while she may seldom use the manual itself, the categories are probably quite similar to the diagnostic categories she has readily available in her mind when she assesses a patient. It was common for both Psychodynamic Psychologists and Biodynamic Psychiatrists to write off the DSM and simultaneously describe (some with more conscious acknowledgment than others) the power of the categories over their thinking.

Dr. Nelson's notions of etiology also have clear implications for how she thinks about treatment. When I asked her to what she attributes the causes of the conditions she treats, she told me, "I'm sort of biopsychosocial. . . . I'm a firm believer in biology. I think there are people who grow up in horrific developmental situations and come out way ahead, and people who can't and that a lot of it is biological. And genetic. And then I think that you know I'm a firm believer in the developmental theory of how we become who we are—all kinds of theories that our social and economic environment also play a huge role." Showing the influence of her psychiatric training, Dr. Nelson describes biology as the most salient of three overlapping etiological concerns—the biological, the psychological, and the social. But resilience, she explains, is both inherited and learned. In noting that there are multiple causal factors in the development of mental illness, Dr. Nelson reaffirms her identity as both a biomedical and psychodynamic practitioner. She feels comfortable using both psychodynamic talk therapy and medication treatments.

Dr. Kane, PhD: Psychodynamic Psychologist

I interviewed Dr. Kane at her home on the Upper East Side of Manhattan on a wintry weekend. I was invited into her living room and seated on a large sofa, where we spent over an hour in conversation. Dr. Kane spoke in dulcet tones and sometimes became lost in her own thoughts, trailing off in the middle of sentences and starting new ideas before finishing others. She was often concerned with making sure to offer the "right" answer and feared she would rethink something after the interview; her worry was about misrepresenting her field rather than being wrong. Dr. Kane was born in the 1960s and grew up in the Northeast. She attended prestigious East Coast schools from college through graduate school and was a psychology intern in New York City in the 1980s. At the time of her interview, Dr. Kane was seeing approximately twenty patients, three of whom were in analysis and three of whom were on some kind of psychotropic medication (prescribed by a psychiatrist). She sees the remainder of her patients for psychodynamic psychotherapy, which means multiple meetings per week (usually two), generally for several years. While twenty patients seems like very few and her practice is smaller than those of most of my interviewees, she sees her three analytic patients twelve hours a week total and the seventeen other patients, whom she sees an average of twice a week, another thirty-four hours, making a total of about forty-six clinical hours (a handful of the seventeen regular therapy patients are in treatment once a week or three times a week).

Dr. Kane's psychology training involved four years of classroom experience, characterized by seminar attendance and extensive reading in psychological theory and treatment approaches; in short, Dr. Kane had a typical experience in a social science graduate program. Her training was predominantly psychodynamically oriented (as opposed to behavioral, which was becoming increasingly popular in the 1980s). As part of her training, Dr. Kane was placed in various clinical settings; psychologists work with patients in clinical settings for most of their graduate career. This was followed by one full year of internship. As a requirement for becoming a PhD, Dr. Kane also had to write and defend a dissertation, demonstrating both a theoretical and a methodological mastery of her field. In order to qualify to be a psychoanalytic candidate at many institutes, psychologists must also complete one year of clinical work beyond their internship in order to be licensed, so unlike her psychiatrist counterparts, Dr. Kane could not go straight from graduate school into analytic training. Psychologists often take more time off between their graduate and postdoctoral work in psychoanalysis than psychiatrists for logistical reasons as well, such as building a client base and saving up enough money since their internships generally pay them far less than what residents make.

Dr. Kane started the five-year training in psychoanalysis (the same postdoctoral training described above for Dr. Nelson) in the late 1990s. She described psychoanalytic training as a natural progression from her psychology training and also as an extension of her deep interests in Freudian theory, in investigations of the mind, and in developing meaningful relationships with patients. When I asked her why she became a therapist and when she made the decision to go to graduate school in psychology, Dr. Kane explained that she knew long before college that she would be a psychologist:

> I have an interest in what motivates people, in people's inner lives. I find it intellectually very stimulating and challenging to make connections between past and present for people. On a more surface level, I enjoy talking to people one-on-one and a type of intimacy that comes out of the relationship is very satisfying in a certain way. . . . I decided very early on, I was about twelve. I took a [psychologically oriented] book off my parents' bookshelf . . . it is funny 'cause it's a book very much of the sixties or seventies, and at twelve you become more open to things and just "oh my goodness, what an interesting way to think about people" and to kind of diagram what's going on. I remember it in the most vague terms . . . but it just caught my attention and it seemed like "oh, well this is an area that I could be thinking about."

Just a minute later, Dr. Kane described an interaction with a patient who came across the same text as an adult, and it was clear that they had bonded over the shared experience. I could see that Dr. Kane had warm feelings about this interchange and that these moments are part of what she loves about her work. She described her choice to enroll in psychoanalytic training as something that happened "pretty early on":

> I can't pinpoint the age but probably even before college, even before I really knew what it was about because when I went on to read more in psychology as a teenager and started to read a little Freud—even though I didn't really understand it—the concepts captured my attention and I was very intrigued by ideas of complexity, of human functioning, and so it was very satisfying to me to read about, to think about, to consider about my parents and people around me and what was going on. It was a passion from early on.

Unlike Dr. Evans, Dr. Sutter, and Dr. Nelson, Dr. Kane did not describe the pragmatic details that influenced her decision to train in psychology or psychoanalysis. For her, it was affection for psychoanalytic ideas and practice, a deep way of exploring functioning, and a fascination with the psyche. She felt not that learning how to be a good talk therapist was a task but rather that it fit naturally with whom she was already, both personally and professionally. This zeal for analytic thinking is clear in how she described what sets psychoanalysis apart from other treatments: "an interest in . . . depth of functioning, and also the interest in creating a long-term relationship or conversation as a mode of treatment."

Dr. Kane's affinity for psychoanalysis is much more than as a treatment paradigm—it is a worldview. When I asked her what she sees as the contribution psychology and psychoanalysis make to society, she indicated that her thinking is very much about the contributions psychoanalytic *theory*, in addition to practice, makes to society:

> It adds a way of understanding and thinking about societal phenomenon . . . for instance, selections from a book I assigned to my psychoanalysis class is on terrorism and violence and selections are written by psychologists and some MD psychoanalysts, but in terms of how to understand, for instance, the upbringing of someone who would become a terrorist or the mind-set of someone who'd become a terrorist or the experience of being dehumanized and then dehumanizing others. I mean that's just a specific example of how I think psychology connects to an understanding of social phenomenon and current events.

Quite differently from Dr. Nelson, Dr. Kane made no mention of reducing symptoms or of mental illness per se. For Dr. Kane, the contribution of her field is much more about thinking about the mind and understanding people.

When I asked her what it is like to be part of the psychoanalytic and psychological communities, she, quite similarly to Dr. Nelson (who described shedding some of her psychiatric identity after doing the psychoanalytic training), told me,

> I identify much more with the psychoanalytic community. I feel that I
> have much more in common in that world than I do with the general psy-
> chological community. Early in my career I would go to American Psy-
> chological Association conventions . . . I identified in that world. But
> as I became more immersed in the psychoanalytic world, those are the
> conferences that I go to—or lectures—so I don't really participate in
> the mainstream world of psychology. Let me add one piece to that,
> which is that I teach . . . psychology students, most of whom have no
> interest in psychoanalysis at all. Even if you don't go on in psychology
> or analysis you can broaden or enrich your perspective [with psycho-
> analytic principles]. . . . So, anyway, my sort of emotional and profes-
> sional affiliations are in the psychoanalytic world, though I have a foot
> in the psychological community.

She explained that it is sometimes difficult to train psychologists whose think-ing is, today, not likely to be analytically oriented; though Dr. Kane feels strongly that psychoanalytic principles are useful for any trainee, the pushback or "kick-back" she describes when she teaches psychodynamic ideals marks her differ-ence from the mainstream psychology community. She explained further that many of her students view psychoanalytic theory as unnecessary for their prac-tices and are actually antagonistic to Freudian ideas about the central role of sexuality in psychological development and adult thinking.

Dr. Kane feels unlike the majority of the psychologists she trains. But when I asked if she sees herself differently from the psychoanalysts who are psychia-trists, like Dr. Nelson, she replied that she thinks she is more likely to think like a Biodynamic Psychiatrist than like a psychologist:

> I actually don't think there's a huge difference in thinking. I think that
> there are, around the periphery, like an MD psychoanalyst might jump
> in more towards medical or diagnostic, DSM diagnostic explanations for
> things. . . . Psychologist analysts may be a little less prone to pigeonhole,
> more open to the broader phenomenon of the patient 'cause our training

is not so diagnostically and bodily—you know, bodily in a literal way. So, I think that's around the periphery, but I think for the most part I'm more likely to think like an MD psychoanalyst than the average psychologist who's not an analyst.

Yet when I asked Dr. Kane directly if she sees tensions between psychologist and psychiatrist analysts, she replied emphatically,

> Yes. Yes. For example, I was at a symposium this weekend . . . and one of the presenters whose presentation was wonderful, he gave some really great case material, he's somebody who I've heard before and respect a great deal. He's an MD psychoanalyst and totally gratuitously in the context of his presentation, he said that MD psychoanalysts are more likely to focus on the body. But he didn't mean literally the body like symptoms or diagnoses, just on patients' experiences of their bodies. And I happened to be sitting, by coincidence, in a row where there were several psychologists and we sort of turned and looked at each other like what the hell is he talking about. . . . It was not accurate and I had no idea why he put that in there. It just didn't even make any sense. . . . I do think that MD psychoanalysts think of themselves at the top of the hierarchy.

Even though Dr. Kane believes that her thinking is aligned with that of Biodynamic Psychiatrists, she clearly feels as though there is some way in which they relegate the Psychodynamic Psychologists to secondary status, and sees their medical training as the factor that allows them to do so. So, she is somewhat caught in between the psychoanalytic world where she is lower in the hierarchy and psychology, a field she no longer feels all that aligned with.

Though the DSM was designed by and for psychiatrists, Dr. Kane does have to think about DSM categories and use them for insurance purposes. When I asked her what the role of DSM is in practice, she chuckled and responded, "Very little." However, in the next breath she said, "I feel *obligated* when first meeting someone to consider DSM because I want to think about whether I *ought* to be referring them for medication, for instance, or whether there's character pathology that I should be taking into account, or thinking about as I approach my work with this person. But beyond the first couple sessions or unless I hear new material as we go that then puts me back to criteria for [something like] depression, I consider it very little ever once I'm amidst a treatment." Given that Dr. Kane is a psychologist and cannot prescribe medications like her Biodynamic counterparts, she describes the obligation as an "ought" feeling that she should refer patients for medications when symptoms are quite severe, when the intensity and/or duration of a patient's symptoms are beyond a tolerable range. When I asked her whom she tends to refer her patients to for medications, she informed me that she would "prefer to refer to fellow analysts," citing with a smile that they "can have a conversation that makes sense and takes into account the dynamics of the patient." Because of that, a Biodynamic Psychiatrist is also less likely to get in the way of the treatment plan or alter the narrative that Dr. Kane and her patient have previously established about the treatment overall, and about the meaning and cause of the patient's symptoms.

Because she refers her patients for medicine, the role of medication in her treatment is certainly a consideration, as Dr. Kane explains:

> I think one role that it sometimes can play is to sort of free up someone from symptoms that couldn't then interfere with their life and that they're freed up actually to focus on other more neurotic issues. I'm not a big medication person, as I'm sure most psychologist analysts are not 'cause I think that sometimes there's a lot of fantasy around medication, a lot of ideas about "well now I'm better" and appreciating sort of the short-term, cut and dry, yes/no aspects of it, as opposed to the actual hard work of an ongoing therapy.

Though Dr. Kane cannot prescribe drugs and only a handful of her patients take them, she makes it clear that, for patients with severe symptoms, she will certainly refer them to a psychiatrist. Dr. Kane is very careful to pay attention to the meaning of medications for her patients, and will discuss, in-depth, how the patient feels about taking medicines. When asked specifically if she considers the prominent role of medication to be problematic for the profession of psychiatry, Dr. Kane shrugged sort of exasperatedly several times as she responded:

> I think it's very problematic and I think it's driven by reasons other than actually what's helpful for patients, such as insurance company reimbursement. . . . This isn't something I've thought about a lot, it's not something I think about a lot, but the American Psychiatric Association, since that's their thing, medication is their thing, you know. It may be a way of protecting the guild essentially, and insuring a livelihood for their members. . . . I think it's a problem for psychiatry in that psychiatrists coming up are not being trained to do very much psychotherapy, and certainly not very much psychodynamic psychotherapy, so I think they're becoming, as I see it, almost robotic in a certain way.

This overreliance on medications is not the same in her profession, but since she teaches analysts in training, many of whom are psychiatrists, Dr. Kane has become familiar with the kind of training psychiatrists have, and feels they sometimes struggle to become good talk therapists when they enter analytic training (as Dr. Nelson corroborates).

Summarizing her thinking quite nicely was Dr. Kane's succinct reply to my question about the etiology of the conditions she treats: "Nature and nurture, biology and environment. Environment including early history, chance . . . I think more about the environmental, more about the nurture." Unlike the Biomedical Psychiatrists, Drs. Evans and Sutter, Dr. Kane's notion of environment focuses on early family life and relationships, even though she makes sure to think about potential biological vulnerabilities as well.

In the chapters to follow, I turn to a focused discussion of many of the issues Drs. Evans, Sutter, Nelson, and Kane raised, with particular attention to the roles of diagnosis, medication, and talk therapy in treatment as well as the experience of practicing in a field dominated by the biomedical model.

Chapter 3

The Promise of "Imperfect Communication" and the "Prison" of Rigid Categorization

The DSM in Practice

Dr. Poplar is a Biomedical Psychiatrist whose residency years spanned the late 1980s. She describes her psychiatry training as "pretty biologically based . . . with some emphasis on family, grief treatments, and interpersonal psychotherapy." Dr. Poplar does not see any patients solely for talk therapy, but she is not strictly a psychopharmacologist; though most of her patients take antidepressants, only ten or so see her for medication management alone. She explained that she tries to "go through everything" when she first meets a patient: "I spend about an hour and a half on the first interview gathering both subjective impressions and their reported history. If there's anything medical, I certainly try to get the medical records, I try to talk to any prior psychiatric caregiver, medication response often points to diagnosis or misdiagnosis. Those are the main things." Her initial encounter with patients is structured and diagnosis is an essential part of her practice. When I asked her specifically about the DSM, Dr. Poplar offered a typically terse but instructive response: "I think it's our main reference tool. We don't have critical lab values and we don't have—it is, in some ways it's not our hardest science—but it's our greatest thinkers, presumably, compiled this in an effort to advance our field. But it's constantly changing . . . this is a work in progress." A practitioner for over thirty years at the time of our interview, a pragmatic clinician, and a student of biomedical psychiatry, Dr. Poplar captured the typical ambiguity and even aloofness I encountered when I asked about the role of the DSM in my interviewees' practice: the DSM is central but imperfect. And the categories within it are seen as largely valid, yet the knowledge in the field is very much in flux.

The clinicians with whom I spoke described the DSM as "the bible," "the big book" (a reference to Alcoholics Anonymous's rulebook), as Strunk and White's classic guidebook for writers, and as "the cookbook." Some used more derogatory language. My questions about the role the DSM plays in their practices elicited a range of visceral reactions, from disgust at the "pigeonholing" of patients to incredulousness at the extent of knowledge and travail involved in its production—often at the same time. It isn't surprising that the practitioners in this study have competing sentiments about the DSM, as it represents all at once the austerity of classification in the biomedical model, the promise of clear communication between practitioners, and an evidence-based model that many in the field of psychiatry have worked toward since even before the biomedical revolution in the 1980s. Notwithstanding the strong feelings about this diagnostic system, which is lauded by some and detested by others, and despite its centrality to the field, it is often written off as simply a "reference tool" and even mocked for what many think is an overstated role in their practice and thinking. It is sometimes seen as "the gold standard," yet often also as a "trap" designed to cast a wider net around patients' experiences.

The DSM as the "Gold Standard"

The most common response practitioners gave to my question about the utility of the DSM was that it organizes thinking. In evidence-based medicine, DSM categories are the foundation of research and practice. Dr. Warren (Biodynamic) explains the crucial role of DSM in research: "You can't really do studies without something like a DSM. You just can't because if some guy out in Kansas is calling something one thing and we don't even have the criteria to validate that it's the same thing, that's ridiculous." In practice, the DSM can serve a similar purpose, as Dr. Troy (Biodynamic) explains,

> I think that what DSM does is that, first of all, it helps us all to speak the same language with the same grounding, and that's huge. Because it allows for some degree of consistency and it allows us as clinicians to communicate. Otherwise it would be very hard. It's an imperfect communication, but at least its communication speaking the same language. So that's one big thing. The other is it helps you conceptualize. . . . Sometimes when a diagnosis is unclear the DSM is actually helpful because if you actually kind of conceptually think of the criteria, it can help certainly clarify what seems like a very confusing patient.

Dr. Troy describes the most basic use of the DSM and its intended purpose—as a system of classification used for clear conceptualization and communication.

As such, the DSM combats many of the critiques of early twentieth century psychiatry, which was unable to provide reliable diagnosis; different practitioners often classified the same patient using different terminology. The lack of shared language left psychiatry open to critiques from supporters of the evidence-based model both within and outside the field. Psychoanalysts were especially attuned to the legitimacy the DSM provides for the field.

Though practitioners were sometimes quick to reject the widespread notion that DSM is the bible of psychiatry, most do believe it's a central guiding text in their field. Dr. Reeve (Biomedical) was clear that she doesn't "think it's a bible." Rather, she says, "it's a guideline." She continued,

> You know, if I'm talking to a colleague and they say oh, I have a depressed patient, then it helps us to be on the same page about what we're talking about. And in research, if you wanna read it, and it's about depressed patients and you sort of assume that there's a certain category of patient that it fits for. But it's descriptive, because in psychiatry I don't have a standard for your blood pressure, I don't have a blood test for most things, so I need something that helps to put a framework on things and that's what DSM does. But you know this is the fourth revised whatever edition, so clearly that is a work in progress also.

The strength of the DSM, my interviewees explained, is in its standardization, which is critical for diagnosis, for treatment, and for validating the legitimacy of those treatments, as well as psychiatry's rightful place as a medical discipline. Discrete categorization is even more important in psychiatry than in other fields where other diagnostic measures can demonstrate the presence or absence of disease. Several of the Biomedical and one of the Biodynamic Psychiatrists described the benefits of brain scanning (fMRI or otherwise) for identifying illness, though largely as a potential future development in the field. Especially in private practice, this technology is not currently practical. The most biomedically oriented of all my interviewees works in a building that has at least one fMRI machine, though she did not mention these kinds of scanning technologies as a routine part of her practice. Furthermore, brain scans have yet to offer clear insights into the etiology, prognosis, or appropriate treatment of mental health troubles.

Dr. Brown (Biodynamic) also described the utility that diagnostic categories and standardization have for validating mental health problems as "real" medical conditions in need of medical treatment. She depicted the DSM as "a useful construct" because, she says, "the problem with psychiatry is that we don't have laboratory tests, so a lot of diagnosis is made descriptively, which is

most unfortunate in certain ways because the meaning of it, in a way, one particular symptom might have multiple meanings, so it's very tricky to just rely
on symptomatology." In the same breath as she critiques the categories in the
DSM, she recognizes that they validate the notion of psychiatry as a medical
field. Dr. Doughty (Biomedical) perhaps most clearly exemplifies the various
competing feelings about the DSM:

> I think we need it. I think even now, and certainly, in the seventies and
> eighties and nineties, you know, psychiatry is not considered on par with
> other medical specialties. Largely because our diagnosis is all what we
> hear, what we ask, what we observe. For the most part, there are no tests
> that you can do. There is no way to validate your findings and so people,
> I think, psychiatrists earlier were using terms very loosely and meaning
> different things by it. I don't think you can have that. I don't think that
> is helpful to the field. I don't think it is helpful to the patients either. If
> five different psychiatrists are going to define depression five different
> ways then you don't know—the treatment becomes meaningless. Or, the
> idea of treatment approach becomes meaningless. . . . The main positive
> is that I think to a large extent psychiatrists know what other psychia-
> trists mean when they use a term. The main negative is that it is some-
> what confining. But maybe it needs to be confining and I think the other
> negative, which may be clearer, is that there is a tendency to pathologize,
> it allows you to pathologize behavior that lots of people would not nec-
> essarily think is an illness.

While she recognizes the DSM promotes a "tendency to pathologize," a common concern I turn to shortly, in general Dr. Doughty clearly captures the link
to validity and reliability offered by a system of discrete diagnoses.

When I asked Dr. Brighton (Psychodynamic) if she found the categories in
the DSM useful, she said, "not really," but then quickly continued:

> You know sometimes you might be a little confused about a picture of
> someone because they're mixed and they have a lot of different things
> going on and it might be a little helpful to go to the manual and look at
> okay, what's OCD? I have a patient who has OCD, ADD, and depression
> and she's borderline character disorder, she's got it all, so because she's
> such a complex picture it's sometimes helpful to just read all of what's
> laid out so you have a clearer reason about why it's so hard. . . . In talk-
> ing to other doctors, in making referrals. It's a quick way of speaking to
> ally professionals . . . I've sent her to a million different people.

Dr. Brighton confirms the use of DSM for organizing thinking, particularly with a complicated case, and for communicating about that case with other practitioners. I was struck by how infrequently practitioners described the DSM in terms of its utility for patients' conceptualizations of their experiences, although I often heard stories of patients who come into a treatment looking for specific medications or diagnoses, as was the case in my conversation with Dr. Halsey (Biodynamic). She explained, "Sometimes the patients want to know a name for whatever they're struggling with," which Dr. Halsey told me "is comforting somehow, and sometimes in a very genuine way. If you are just overwhelmed and you don't know what's going on and somebody calls it anxiety disorder and then you read it and you say 'Oh yeah, that sounds good,' that can be comforting." Much as diagnostic categories help practitioners organize their thinking, patients, who are often confused or upset by their symptoms, want a clear explanation for their experiences. Sometimes this is difficult for practitioners who have to combat misinformation their patients find online or incorrect self-diagnoses rooted in ideas from friends and family, but practitioners generally told me access to information is positive, as long as it is accurate.

When I asked her about the DSM, Dr. Ferris (Biodynamic) chuckled, as if to say "of course you're asking about that silly thing," a surprisingly common reaction. Like Dr. Brighton, she conveyed the utility of the DSM in clarifying and making distinctions. She explained that she "was trained using the DSM," as were the majority of the psychiatrists I spoke with (with the exception of the three most senior), so she uses it as she was taught to, as the guiding framework for diagnosis. Yet she worries about accuracy:

> I think about categories. Sometimes it's harder to make distinctions in a diagnosis if you know someone has a delusional disorder versus depression, delusional depression versus sometimes other psychotic disorders, schizophrenia. So, I have to think about it and I will refer to my DSM if I'm trying to make a distinction between those because there might be, there would be a difference in medication that you would chose possibly or if someone had bipolar disorder or a schizoaffective disorder you might chose differently medication-wise. But you know otherwise, in terms of Axis II or nonpsychotic disorders, I don't think I refer very much to DSM.[1] It doesn't, other than, I think I sort of formulate much more as an analyst in terms of defenses and predominant defensive style and predominant character style.

Dr. Ferris points to a common use of the DSM for her colleagues—with difficult cases or those that seem not to fit easily identifiable categories. In order to be careful to get a diagnosis "right," my interviewees describe using DSM categories particularly when a patient's symptoms seem as though they could fall under multiple diagnoses or when they are uncommon. Dr. Ferris expressly consults the DSM only for unclear cases. She also explained the importance of accurate diagnosis for proper prescribing, although I was told repeatedly that most practitioners tend to use a handful of medications they feel most comfortable with to treat a wide range of conditions related to anxiety and depression. Several practitioners noted they feel most at ease using medications they know well, so it is important to rule out, for example, bipolar disorder, before prescribing an antidepressant, but once a practitioner establishes that a patient is experiencing some form of depression or anxiety, the specific diagnosis will likely not dramatically change the treatment.

At first, I was struck by how rarely practitioners (particularly psychiatrists) said they directly consulted the DSM, as most practitioners say they use it only for tough cases. But I learned that what I originally thought was an indication of the periphery of the DSM is actually a clue that most of the time practitioners don't *need* it; relying on their memory of the classifications from training, they rarely need to consult the physical manual. My realization of the extent to which the DSM model is internalized came when Dr. Warren (Biodynamic), who had just moments earlier talked about how little she uses formal diagnostic checklists, herself realized the extent of her diagnostic thinking:

> The funny part is like half the time I'm not thinking this is DSM, I'm just thinking oh, let's get the symptoms of this and find out where we are on this, but *it is* DSM. . . . So I do think it's important, but . . . it's so depressing to me how many people just use checklists these days. . . . There's a danger to that especially with teenagers I find because they break up with a boyfriend or girlfriend and one day they're like the most depressed-looking kid in the universe and then if you saw them forty-eight hours later, and they're with their friends, they're fine . . . if you just use the DSM without good clinical judgment it can really be a joke.

In hinting at some of the troubles with the DSM that I describe shortly, Dr. Warren epitomizes the difficult position in which many practitioners find themselves: they are highly critical of the same diagnostic categories that they have been socialized to see and to think of as real entities. Dr. Lewis's (Biodynamic) almost instinctual response to my question about the role of the DSM in her practice was, "I hate it." A somewhat raucous laughter accompanied the words as they left her lips. She continued,

When I teach I always tell the residents do not use the DSM as the text-book of psychiatry. It's a useful research tool, it's a useful communication tool and it's a useful billing tool. So what I do is I get an honest DSM diagnosis, I do, in part because I need to see clearly of what I'm thinking about treating. In part because I want to get the number I can give the patient who will then submit it to the insurance and within that I try to use a code that's nicer than a less nice code if I can and a code that I can memorize easily. And I don't remember the day when apart from my last board exam that I touched a DSM. I just look for the number in my little book. There are two copies somewhere.

As Dr. Lewis turned toward the bookcase where there were indeed two editions of the DSM (as there were in almost all the psychiatrists' offices I visited), I processed her dismissive tone regarding the manual, and Dr. Warren's words, "It *is* DSM," played in my head. While the existence of physical copies of the DSM in practitioners' offices was a clear sign of the presence of the diagnostic model in the field, what was more striking was the way in which practitioners talked about *not* needing to directly consult the DSM on a regular basis; training, particularly for the Biodynamic and Biomedical practitioners, means learning the categories well enough in psychiatry training not to need to consult the DSM regularly. Practitioners took my question about the role of the DSM in their practices literally—if they don't generally consult the manual, they considered it to play a minor (or no) role, but most of them underestimated the extent to which many years of training to think of patients in terms of DSM categories colors their thinking. I suspect this is one of the underlying factors in the almost predictable laughter that accompanied our conversations around the DSM.

In her explanation of the major changes in the field since her training, Dr. Clarendon (Biomedical), who trained in the 1980s, confirms that psychiatry training is increasingly tied to DSM categories:

Training, it's just gotten to be much more about identifying disorders according to the DSM classification. And there is much less attention paid to fundamental, as I see it anyway, the fundamental psychopathology to really sort of the philosophy that underlies the clinical interaction. When I was in residency people really talked about . . . that fundamental question of how you can really know what it is a patient's experiencing. What is it that makes a belief a delusional belief as opposed to some other kind of belief? My sense is that there is not the same attention paid to that kind of thing, and that it's much more about recognition of symptoms and classification symptoms and the DSM is a major guide. I mean my complaint it's the old person's complaint that the younger generation isn't as thoughtful or as smart as we were.

While Dr. Clarendon jokes about the "old person's complaint," she levies a significant critique of the emphasis on diagnosis and the general way residents are trained in biomedical programs.

Psychodynamic Psychologists, who are not trained to use the DSM or to think particularly categorically, and who cannot prescribe medications, tend to think of its utility in fairly basic terms. And like older Biodynamic Psychiatrists, they were much less likely to reference medications at all in their discussion of DSM given that they either cannot or do not prescribe medications. Dr. Butler's (Psychodynamic) description of the DSM was much like those of her colleagues: "Well, other than what you put on the insurance form, which you know again, that's a whole lot in itself, dealing with insurance companies. But you know I think DSM is a rough and ready tool. In the beginning, it can be useful just to assess what you're dealing with and the degree of severity, and is this person a danger to themselves? But beyond that, as you get more into the work, I don't really think about it very much." Diagnostic categories serve practitioners in various ways, by (1) helping to organize their thinking when presented with complex human emotions and experiences; (2) allowing clear communication between practitioners, a kind of shared language for discussing patients' experiences; and (3) allowing patients to receive reimbursement from insurance companies.

However, my interviewees also described DSM categories as restrictive—even as a form of bondage. Perhaps more than any other topic we covered, the DSM represents a point of tension. It was in Dr. Mill's (Biodynamic) words that I first recognized a recurring sentiment about the DSM. She described an instance in which she had to take a board recertification exam in psychiatry:

So, recently, I had to study for a test on DSM. . . . It's irritating, it can be a real pain in the ass, but I remember the pleasure or the enjoyment of the fact that somebody, somewhere put all this work into kind of sorting this stuff out, and it's meaningful. It's actually useful. It's not *the* answer. It's not the end-all. But it's another one of the tools we have and it always reminds me, "hey, this is a good tool." So, does it always play a role [in my practice]? Absolutely. Is it always the number one role? It's always in the top. I think there may be a psychology/psychiatry difference there because . . . I imagine they [psychologists] may not use DSM or at least in the way that I might as a tool to steer things, to help organize a lot of information. A meaningful way to start with, to begin with and then you rule things out, but I do believe it's helpful as a guide. . . . I mean it doesn't contain everything. It doesn't capture everything about a person. . . . I think of it as something sort of plastic, meaning that I can use it the way I want to. So, I know the criteria. Say major depressive episode equals five of nine symptoms for more than two weeks, but I don't particularly get too fussy about whether they've got four or five or whether it's fourteen days or ten days.

Dr. Mill presents the central quandary related to practicing in a diagnostic model for practitioners who are trained in talk therapy, especially psychodynamic psychotherapy or psychoanalysis: it is a guidebook with significant merits but also an excessively rigid handbook that seems to overstep its place in practice and wield excessive power over the field. Dr. Mill was clear that a good practitioner *shouldn't* use the DSM as anything beyond a set of guidelines.

The DSM as a "Trap": The Dangers of Diagnosis

While all but two of the practitioners (older psychoanalysts) I interviewed pointed to clear utilities of the DSM, almost all were also readily able to describe what they see as dangers of the manual and of diagnostic thinking more generally. Most worry about the overly rigid use of DSM categorization, particularly when they feel it represents, or is taught to students as, *the* way of thinking about the range of human emotion and experience. One of the reasons it's often difficult to tell how practitioners truly feel about the DSM is because the widely agreed-upon strength of the DSM for organizing practitioners' thinking is precisely what most of my interviewees also mention when asked about problems with the DSM model. Consider this interchange I had with Dr. Sutter (Biomedical) about psychiatry being, in her words, "DSM driven":

Dr. S: You know I think it is. And I don't think that's bad. I don't think my practice is un-DSM-related. I think about it and I have one on my desk and I pull it out regularly to look at and put numbers down and stuff, but it's just a little too simplistic. It reduces people.

DS: If you think about issues that you have with DSM, is there anything that comes to mind readily, problems that you associate with it?

Dr. S: Just that it's sort of cookbooky and doesn't tell you that much about a person.

DS: And what do you think are the greatest strengths DSM?

Dr. S: That it's cookbooky.

DS: The same thing?

Dr. S: Yeah, that everyone knows what major depression means and that when you read a study and it says, "The people in the study were diagnosed with major depression recurrent," you know who they are. When it says, "They didn't have substance abuse or they didn't have borderline personality," you just know who those people are and then you could sort of think of your own patients.

Dr. Sutter was clear about the strength of the "cookbooky" approach—practitioners can follow the instructions and wind up with a proper diagnosis, much the way one can add the just the right ingredients and wind up with cake batter. But she and many other interviewees also alluded to problems associated with reducing people to the sum of their symptoms. For this reason, Dr. Butler (Psychodynamic) explained that DSM categories are useful only "up to a point": "They're kind of static. I mean, they're not developmental, they're a kind of labeling, a kind of box into which you fit somebody and I think some of the categories don't really, aren't particularly illuminating or useful in terms of treatment . . . you can't really pigeonhole people that neatly." Though Dr. Butler and others clearly believe it's problematic to compartmentalize patients and worry that diagnoses become fixed lenses through which practitioners see their patients, they use the DSM nonetheless.

Like many of her colleagues, Dr. Clarendon (Biomedical) told me she "hates" the DSM, which is particularly intriguing given her medical training and her overwhelmingly biomedical practice:

> I hate it because I think it has, because it's so front and center. It introduced a sort of reductionistic thinking into psychiatry that has crowded out a more skeptical view of what it is we are actually seeing, what it is we are actually treating, and I feel that that's much more of the kind of residency program and the kind of training that I went through rather than what current residents are getting. So, for example, when I went through training there were certainly competing views of how to understand what the patient was experiencing. Obviously the psychoanalytic was one way of understanding it. There was the neurobiological way of understanding it. There was the family systems way of understanding it, and it was felt to be a legitimate area of inquiry to think about other ways to classify the business of psychiatry. So, there were the classifications from the early part of the twentieth century. . . . Paul McHugh at Hopkins published a book, which I think is a wonderful book called *The Perspec-*

tives of Psychiatry, in which he described the different kind of way of sorting out patients and I just feel that the DSM, because of the ease of which it can be taught, has assumed a prominence in training and our conception of what constitutes psychiatric illness that it really isn't justified by the science or by the history.

Dr. Clarendon, like many of her colleagues, describes that what she finds useful in the DSM is precisely what she hates about it. It offers order and clarity at the expense of alternate ways of thinking. Some form of the term "reductionism" appeared across a range of interviews, and a number of the doctors I interviewed were quick to point out that the DSM model pushes them toward thinking about disorder rather than deeper analysis of their patients' experiences. In Dr. Clarendon's description is also a crucial reference to her training. She learned psychodynamic principles, so even though she still practices as a Biomedical Psychiatrist, she thinks deeply about patients' experiences and has another lens through which she can critique the diagnostic model.

The "lumping" effect of DSM diagnosis was one of the problems my interviewees most often associated with biomedical psychiatry. Here, Dr. Elm (Biomedical) denigrates the strict use of the DSM because it ignores nuance and difference:

> All this diagnostic criteria, it's barely useful when you're looking at a complex person, and it doesn't help you understand what's really going on. It lumps a bunch of people together who look similar, but may not be and it doesn't even—it barely helps you even medication-wise at this point. So, all of a sudden everyone who's in this diagnosis gets the same medicine as the people in this diagnosis. That's because what's going on in the brain is probably similar, even though the presentation is different. So, I find the diagnostic criteria not useful and now with what's going on with the DSM-5, I'm actually feeling very depressed.

When I pressed Dr. Elm as to her "depression" about DSM-5, she told me it's because "they're continuing to fight about concepts that feel more political to me than scientific." Dr. Gold (Biodynamic) was also highly critical of the unquestioning use of the DSM, which she notes is part of what upholds the biomedical model: "In a sense, because some people take it literally and use it, it's great for the insurance companies because maybe you should be on medication and be seen once a month—why do you have to see them three times a week or four times a week? And it's a political thing too, the biological people if you write the manual then you can claim that's what the treatment modalities are, so there are power struggles and politics involved there. I think it's most unfortunate that it shifted over so far biological." This by-the-book mentality and the support of institutional forces such as insurance companies and the powerful people in the field, whom Dr. Gold refers to as "the biological people," lead to what was the most often cited problem with the DSM and the diagnostic model more broadly: the potential for overdiagnosis. The sense that the DSM is partisan rather than strictly a clinical or research tool offended a number of my inter-viewees, but most of all the narrow lens—one that favors the medical model and thereby upholds the medicalization of the categories these practitioners treat—is what practitioners told me is their greatest concern. Dr. Hart (Biomedical) explained the core issue with the DSM, which she says is that it "seems to help structure and organize what a psychiatrist does, and make sense of it, but," she says, "when I think of patients, for example, that I treat, the depression, they're all gonna have the same code and they are very, very different indi-viduals." Dr. Morris (Biomedical) is likewise concerned about the potential to "lose track of the person inside the illness, and [to] treat illness instead of the person inside the illness." This focus on diagnosis, many practitioners explained, is linked to sometimes-problematic ideas about what illness is and what causes it.

Conceptual Problems with the DSM and Etiological Fallacies

Dr. Gold (Biodynamic), who was in her seventies at the time of our interview, was one of the most critical of the DSM of all my interviewees. She trained long before psychoanalysis fell out of favor and has clear allegiances to the psycho-dynamic model; she is the closest resemblance of a psychiatrist in the Freudian era of anyone I spoke with. She described the DSM as an attempt at a formal representation of the biomedical model:

> There are some people who call themselves experts on the DSM, which is unfortunate. It's a little bit like—I mean it has certain built in assump-tions that the sum of knowledge about psychiatry and what happens in patients' minds is condensed into DSM-IV, which it isn't really. It's a little bit like, I'm trying to think of—you know when you have an icon on your computer screen that represents something and you call it the icon? That's DSM-IV and its correspondence to what's really behind it or what it's sup-posed to deal with in terms of a body of information, has really nothing, has no bearing.

Dr. Gold is troubled by the misconception that the DSM represents the wide range of human experience and that anyone would specialize in diagnosis.

Though this was not a widely shared sentiment, it is representative of a larger concern about the conceptualization of patients as their DSM diagnoses.

DSM-5 was in construction during the time of my early interviews and was released before the end of my final interview. As such, I asked practitioners how they would feel about adding new categories to the DSM and offered them some examples of conversations around the time of the DSM-5 working groups. Compulsions such as gambling, video gaming, and shopping as well as a potential move to dimensional (and away from strictly categorial) diagnoses were of particular interest to the general public and to many practitioners at the time. I was less interested in my interviewees' opinions on which disorders ought to make it into the new DSM than I was about their broader ideas about etiology and the purpose of diagnosis. As such, I asked Dr. Lewis (Biodynamic) how she would feel about adding compulsive buying or shopping addiction to the DSM, to which she replied,

> That's exactly why I don't like DSM because compulsive buying has many completely diverse and unconnected sources. And it can have different meanings. You may be a compulsive buyer because you hate your husband who's extremely wealthy and you want to screw him, for instance. You can be a compulsive buyer because you feel empty inside and bored. You can be a compulsive buyer because you're envious and you want to get what your friend has. You can do it because you're bipolar and you're manic and you can't control it. You can, you know, be using buying as assuaging your psychological distress of some other source than what I said. Some of those that I said are mostly personality disorders. So, it's crazy. It's just like if I put fever as a term for medicine. Fever I mean yeah, hello, why? And there's a category in medicine of fever of unknown origin, that's a very decent category that tells you that you need to investigate why is there a fever and sometimes you might not find out but it can be an indication of something we don't know. But it's, I hate it. As you tell me my blood pressure goes up from 90 to 120.

Dr. Lewis laughed as she described her rising blood pressure, but she was clearly not joking at her annoyance at the overreliance on a nosology that she feels offers little insight into etiology. Dr. Lewis indicated that a diagnosis should lead only to deeper inquiry as to the source of the illness.

Practitioners often indicated that one of the most significant problems with the DSM is that while it traps people into thinking that everyone fits into a category, it doesn't necessarily have a link to etiology or treatment, as Dr. Evans (Biomedical) explains:

I mean I think the problems are that you know it's a conceptual problem . . . kind of a prison of the DSM, it's a criticism of the fact that we
have created these categories and are trying to stick people who have vari-
ations, conditions in these categories but we haven't quite defined what
a condition is. The DSM in the beginning says this is how we define
mental illness. Interestingly enough, I bet no other area of medicine says
the same, says diagnosis of an illness does not constitute grounds for
treatment. What the hell does that mean? But that's how certain we are
about whether something's an illness or not. It's a very honest statement.
People miss that. It's in the first page of the preface. People miss that all
the time. Nobody ever reads that.

Dr. Evans references here the disclaimer by the APA that the DSM makes no
assumptions about etiology (see chapter 1), nor does it make claims about appropriate types of treatment for the various disorders it classifies. Yet Dr. Evans
also indicates that the DSM has taken on a life of its own as practitioners, she
argues, tend to ignore the proviso on etiology and treatment and assume that
the conditions in the manual are treatable, often using medications. Dr. Evans
also calls out an uncertainty about the proper treatment approach in psychiatry
in comparison to other fields of medicine.

Dr. Brighton (Psychodynamic) described what my interviewees see as the
overarching problem with the manual, when she said it misses "the whole person
in terms of how is a character put together." She questioned, "What's the history
of trauma, and does the person know who they are?" As such, she described the
DSM model as deficient in the very ideas central to psychoanalysis.

It lacks any kind of description of etiology. How is a patient becoming OCD?
Okay, so you can say if a patient looks like this, this, and this she's got OCD,
but it tells you nothing about how to really treat that because it's talking
about it only in terms of treating it with medication. So, there's nothing to
help you treat those symptoms using an understanding, an etiology of OCD,
the etiology of substance abuse. . . . It would be lovely to have something
descriptive about etiology, typical patterns, family patterns, whatever.

For Psychodynamic Psychologists, who are always concerned with the psychological etiology of the conditions they treat, the DSM provides very little information useful to how they practice.

Psychologists and psychiatrists alike described the inability of the DSM to
really offer any insight beyond clustering symptoms, and specifically its inability to get at explain the derivation of the multitude of conditions they treat. Consider Dr. Clarendon's (Biomedical) description of the problems with the DSM:

The problem with DSM is that it does not address causation. Really at all. It does not, put it this way, it doesn't really provide a coherent frame of understanding of the neurobiological underpinnings of psychiatric disorders, and I think that using the DSM, it's sometimes, or we often lose sight of the fact that it's a way of providing common language to describe patients that we are seeing. But in and of itself it doesn't have any particular scientific validity, and the groupings, the way that the illnesses are grouped really have a lot to do with how historically we have, especially the Kraepelinian split between the mood and the schizophrenic disorders. And that may actually, I think, it will end up having less and less relevance to the treatments that are ultimately helpful for these disorders. So, what I don't like about it is the fact that I think it's often regarded as telling you more about the patient or more about how to treat the patient than it actually does.

Dr. Clarendon struggles a little to clearly explain what she sees as the overarching trouble with the DSM, which is that it almost deludes practitioners into thinking it offers more answers than it does. She also alludes to the idea that DSM categories somewhat arbitrarily split certain kinds of disorders from others in a way that may not actually help with treatment. In other words, she and others describe a sense of randomness associated with the ways the DSM both lumps symptoms together and splits certain conditions from others. As a research tool, its intended purpose, the DSM offers a promise of shared knowledge, but in clinical practice, my interviewees note, it can serve to limit thinking at the same time as it organizes it. And again, while the DSM reminds us it makes no claims about etiology, Dr. Clarendon, like many of the other practitioners I interviewed, is clear that many people ignore that basic fact in addition to assuming that the DSM depicts valid, real entities, rather than social constructions—categories created by people who carve up the world in particular ways. Practitioners note a significant tension between the DSM's claim of etiological neutrality but its use as a tool of biomedical psychiatry and I heard repeatedly of concerns that the reification of the conditions the DSM describes may actually work against the goal of gaining a clear picture of patients' troubles.

External Pressures: Insurance and Pharma

Beyond standardization and organizing thinking, the most often mentioned practical uses of the DSM were for insurance reimbursement and for accurately prescribing medication. The DSM is often described as something of a necessary evil. Use of the DSM for making sure to choose an appropriate medication is generally described as one of its positive attributes related to its use as a heuristic tool. Descriptions about the DSM's ties to insurance companies are less favorable. My interviewees described the use of the DSM for insurance reimbursement in a range of ways: mostly as a neutral document used for practical purposes and occasionally as an icon that ties a corrupt industry to their practice. Dr. Morris (Biomedical) offers the common, somewhat detached, unemotional description of DSM as a useful tool, what she calls a "resource," but she says "other times, it's just like a checklist for the insurance company, like to make sure that I've got the right coding and stuff like that." Dr. Morris generally described the DSM as "the cookbook," which she says, "gives you the recipe for each diagnosis," yet she "wouldn't say it's a big presence in the office except to get something to write down for the insurance." In terms of whether she finds DSM categorizations useful, Dr. Halsey (Biodynamic), told me, "Clinically, not really. They're useful to be able to make the diagnosis and to put it in the insurance forms and again these are insurance forms whenever the patient uses the insurance. If they don't, I generally have a very general mood disorder NOS,[2] and it just stays that way and we don't really go too much into the diagnosis." Most of my interviewees mentioned insurance as a reason to use the DSM only slightly less often than they described it as a way to organize thinking, although the frequency with which particularly psychiatrists referred to the DSM as a tool for organizing their thinking, but then wrote it off as a tool of the insurance companies, left me with a sense that the use by insurance companies, while a tangible and often frustrating part of practice, may offer something of a scapegoat for critiques of a manual that is more central to practice than many practitioners would like to admit.

Dr. Elm was the most critical of the DSM of any of the Biomedical Psychiatrists. She described the biggest shift she's seen since her training (in the 1970s) as "the impact of the change in health care on the practice of psychiatry." She explained further, "The increase in regulation of how we're supposed to function has impacted practice, whether it's from documenting things for HIPPA or electronic health record type things, or if one is involved with managed care in any way." Even clinicians like Dr. Elm, who is not an insurance provider, explained their frustrations: "I experience many hours a week more at work having to do with getting prescriptions authorized. . . . I can't just prescribe what I think is right. I have to think about what's going to be covered, I have to beg the insurance companies to do it, so there's a lot more time spent in administrative things that actually have no function other than procrastinating payment for services." Here, Dr. Elm was referencing trouble with coverage for medication, which requires particular diagnostic codes. Practitioners often have to defend their diagnoses to insurance companies or choose carefully to make sure their patients receive reimbursement for office visits as well as payment for medications.

When seeking to help patients with reimbursement, all practitioners have to deal with insurance companies, as Dr. Reeve (Biomedical) does. She explains the link between the use of the DSM and insurance reimbursement in referring to a scenario in which she was treating a child whose parent came in for "parent guidance": "You know, how do I put a [DSM] code on that that helps them to get some money back? But sometimes the parenting issues or lack of knowledge about parenting is the reason that there are things going on, and Mom might be depressed because she feels incompetent or whatever so it's a relevant issue but there's really no good way to code that." Dr. Reeve recognizes that a DSM code is necessary for a parent to receive some reimbursement for treatment, but the manual is limiting in this regard because many of the usual troubles patients present with don't fit the DSM model of illness. Similarly, Dr. Hart (Biomedical) uses the DSM to figure out what she's "dealing with," but also because she has to provide the DSM diagnosis to the patient "so that they can get reimbursed through insurance." While she appeared annoyed as the word "insurance" left her mouth, Dr. Hart's tone brightened somewhat as she explained that there are "some people who don't want to submit to insurance." While most people in Dr. Hart's practice do want to be able to submit forms for reimbursement, especially since she is a psychiatrist and therefore commands some of the highest fees in the field, she explained that when patients don't need or want to submit to insurance, it's "actually kind of nice" for her because she doesn't "feel constrained into having to plug somebody into a diagnostic category." In other words, when insurance reimbursement is off the table, there is more freedom to creatively interpret symptoms or simply not to worry about categorization as intensely. Unfortunately, that means patients with the greatest financial resources seem the easiest to treat.

Many of the practitioners I spoke with were also clear that the DSM is a tool of the pharmaceutical industry whose representatives influenced its production. Dr. Stanley (Biomedical), for instance, reminded me that "the pharmaceutical industry had a huge part in DSM." She explained further, "They influence the DSM committees. A lot of people that sat on those committees were high ranking in the pharmaceutical industry. That is *so* unethical." Pharmaceutical companies benefit from psychiatrists' belief in biological etiology and their use of the DSM, since it reinforces the notion that treatment with mediation is the most useful option. Dr. Halsey (Biodynamic) also described more nefarious routes of influence by pharmaceutical companies on psychiatric practice: "I'm a consultant for a publication and they need people who are not paid by the drug companies, and it's very hard to find psychiatrists or child psychiatrists if you look into all the departments, the big heads and say you can't be getting any money from the drug companies . . . so, I mean, that's the moment—where do you turn to find people who are not influenced by the enterprise?" In other words, when looking for psychiatrists to publish with or for reliable information about psychopharmacological practice and medication efficacy, it's difficult for Dr. Halsey to know whom to trust and which research hasn't been influenced by the pharmaceutical industry.

The Rigidity of Diagnostic Categories and Flexibility as a Sign of Prestige

With the exception of the four Biomedical Psychiatrists who have the most psychopharmacological practices, all my interviewees pointed to the rigidity of diagnostic categories as something to be leery of; they described the need for the DSM to be used as a guide by a discerning doctor. All the Psychodynamic Psychologists and many of the Biodynamic Psychiatrists expressed concerns that echo Dr. Adams's (Psychodynamic) statement that despite being considered discrete, the categories "bleed into each other." She continued,

> For example, you see a person where there's a strong family history of mood disorder, let's say, and they have children. Let's say there's been suicide on one or both sides of the family. There's been maybe some manic episodes and depressive episodes. And they have a child, and the child has ADHD. Very common situation. Is that ADHD? Is that some kind of general physiological or biochemical disequilibrium that's expressing itself this way, in this generation, or at this age, but it'll change later? I find that whatever that is that's being transmitted biologically can take different forms and at different ages. . . . So, I think it's a waste of time to worry too much about what is the diagnosis, but rather to be sort of open to seeing how it evolves and what's needed at a particular time. . . . Even in medicine [at large], I think good doctors are open to the possibility that what their patient has is something that doesn't neatly fit into any category.

In Dr. Adams's words, there is not only a description of the importance of a wait-and-see approach to diagnosis, but also the notion that being a "good doctor" is bound up in being careful not to take anything at face value and in being able to think flexibly both in the moment and about the future. This was a common sentiment for the Psychodynamic Psychologists who generally do not have any formal training in DSM diagnosis. At the same time, Dr. Adams speaks in diagnostic categories; whether major depressive disorder or bipolar disorder or ADHD, these are DSM categories that she talks about as entities she's on the hunt for.

Perhaps more than any other consequence of the centrality of DSM categorization, my interviewees discussed the dangers of diagnosis for students, especially, psychiatry, as Dr. Dean (Biodynamic) does here: "Someone who has one symptom may fit into a different diagnostic category. Just because you chose one ultimately doesn't mean he doesn't fit into the other one too. . . . I think that in some ways it prevents our students from getting to know the patient sometimes because they're so busy trying to accumulate symptoms so that they can figure out what the diagnosis is sometimes at the expense of finding out more about the patient. DSM ultimately, I think, is more of a research tool, which is valuable, than it is a great clinical tool." Dr. Dean pointed out that the DSM can be dangerous for clinicians in training because they learn to classify people's symptoms, rather than really attend to the humanity of the patient. Dr. Troy (Biomedical) describes a similar concern that residents are often pushed to memorize classificatory schemes. Instead, she says, she teaches concepts:

> I mean I actually teach [the criteria] all the time to the residents. . . . I say to them "your reading instructions are: do not read the criteria. So next week we are going to go over psychotic disorders, your job is to go home and not read the criteria, do no read what's in the box." In the old DSM it [the symptoms] used to be in a box. In 5 they took the box out. I say, "don't read the box! Read everything else around the box because what's around the box is actually what is the concept behind the disease. This is why we think these symptoms have all ended up in one category." It tells you about the course of the illness, it tells you about the very nature of it. . . . If you have that concept in your head then you don't need to do the mathematical check box system, so that's why I think the DSM is very handy for that. Unfortunately, most people don't use it that way. So, our residents would all buy, when they start their residency, that spiral bound copy volume and I say to them you have just wasted twenty-five bucks because this is a laundry list, why would you want this? You don't want this. Buy the text.

Dr. Troy explained with frustration that residents are often told to memorize symptoms and diagnostic categories without attending to what she considers the more important "concept of the illness." The "spiral bound" text to which Dr. Troy refers is an abridged version of DSM that summarizes the diagnostic categories almost solely based on symptomatology and ignores the information about the course of the illness and the logic of the diagnostic category that Dr. Troy feels is so important for understanding patients. At the same time as Dr. Troy critiques the use of shortcuts for understanding people, she also reinforces the biomedical model by looking to the DSM for information about prognosis and even etiology. Her critique of the overreliance on symptomatology represents her feelings about a need to think beyond symptoms, but she supports the idea that DSM descriptions are helpful. And they are valuable, especially because, as Dr. Brooks (Biomedical) explained, "as a trainee, you're sort of barraged by stuff, and complex emotions and behaviors." DSM categories help residents make sense of the symptoms patients present with.

Although the DSM helps especially early career practitioners organize their thinking, it can also distract from more creative and alternate ways of thinking about the human condition. Dr. Elliot (Biodynamic) explains both sides of the argument when she describes the DSM as a framework that allows psychiatric residents to learn how to understand their patients, but she also confirms the notion that a surface-level understanding of patients can be damaging for treatment:

> My own, emotional response—I feel that it's a good sort of frame for beginners, but it really limits people's understanding to follow DSM totally. I sort of feel that it's important to know about what's in there, but it often does not serve when you're really trying to understand the individual person. . . . I'm thinking about this in terms of young psychiatrists. It may limit the clinician's understanding of the person in depth and the empathy with what the person experienced. And sometimes the young clinicians are so worried about how to put the person in the category that they can't listen to what the person is saying about their life. Yeah, I know they have a thing for extreme stress, but when you hear the story of someone who's living in poverty, whose apartment burned down, who has drug addicts outside the door and all of that, stressful environment, sometimes it's more important to hear the individual's story, their life, ya know.

Dr. Stanley (Biomedical), who describes her residency as having been very psychodynamic, most clearly illustrates both the sense of being trapped by the categories and of struggling to teach residents that there's more to people than the DSM would lead them to believe. Dr. Stanley doesn't see the DSM as the bible of psychiatry, but, she says, "I feel constrained by it. I feel more like it ties my hands, I feel more like it is a bit of the bondage book, I don't know." She laughed at the allusion to a sadomasochistic relationship with the DSM, but her demeanor turned more serious as she repeated that she "feels constrained by it." She continued, "I train my residents, I say you never see anything that exactly fits the DSM. These are models to describe very complex symptoms and you're never going to see anything that is exactly perfect. And I teach personality disorders so I always tell them to, you know, look underneath it. If someone has depression and is not getting better after years of treatment and ECT and five different meds, why aren't they getting better? Or what character pathology do they have? So I don't see it as my bible." When Dr. Warren (Biodynamic) describes the benefits of the DSM model for organizing practitioners' thinking early on in a treatment, she also references the dangers of circumventing a deeper assessment of patients and, in this way, points out the different approaches to using the DSM categories:

> You know, it's interesting. DSM does play a role in my practice . . . especially when I'm taking a step back on an initial consultation, or if a patient comes in with a new description of symptoms I haven't heard about before. . . . When I'm sitting with someone and they're talking about their week and something that happened, their conversation with their mother, I'm not thinking about DSM or whatever. And I think it's interesting because I use DSM of course, but it's funny I think to some degree I think the more clinical practice you have—and maybe, if I was a psychopharm person, I would do this differently—but like I'm not sitting there ticking off five out of nines all the time.[3]

A recurrent theme in my interviews with psychoanalysts was the notion that "more clinical practice" makes the DSM categories less central; in other words, a seasoned practitioner shouldn't need to think so categorically. Many of my interviewees described the rigidity and the emphasis on fitting patients into categories as a necessary part of learning, but one that good practitioners grow out of.

Pointing out that there is much more to their practice than assessing symptoms is also a way Biodynamic Psychiatrists distinguish themselves from the "psychopharm person." Dr. Warren explained that she needs the DSM only if something novel arises—if a patient presents with a symptom she hasn't seen before. It is "good clinical judgment" that protects practitioners from making mistakes and, as some called it, "pigeonholing" their patients. While some practitioners seem to find the categories validating, there is a simultaneous prestige in being able to use DSM categories flexibly, particularly for the psychoanalysts, who often described their ability to be discerning and careful not to compartmentalize their patients as one of the benefits of their psychoanalytic training. This sense of pride in being unlikely to use the DSM in a rigid manner became clear early on. Dr. Gold (Biodynamic; one of the oldest of my interviewees) has been in practice for over fifty years. She seemed to regard my question about diagnosis almost as something beneath her, and she somewhat proudly told me, "I could do a clinical evaluation without having to ask them any questions. Appearance, attitude, behavior, speech, affect, sensory perception. You can evaluate all those things without having to ask very much in the way of specific questions. You can do a whole mental status exam just by sitting down and listening to them." Dr. Gold previously told me in a joking tone that psychopharmacology does not interest her. "Let's face it," she says, "writing prescriptions for pills for people that you see for fifteen minutes. I mean, it's a great way of making money, but it isn't very interesting. If you're interested in making money that's what you do and there are a lot of people doing that but it's not very challenging." Dr. Gold sets herself apart from Biomedical Psychiatrists by pointing out what she sees as surface-level practices of other practitioners who are much more wedded to the biomedical model whether it is strictly in terms of diagnosis or in terms of prescribing medications as a vocation. Dr. Ferris (Biodynamic) explains, in a much less derogatory description, that most practitioners today may not even know what the psychodynamic approach truly is:

> I think, you know, that probably if psychiatrists do not—either through experience or through education—have much to do with analytic treatment or people who have been treated analytically, or colleagues who are analysts, they may not fully appreciate what the difference [between them and an analyst] is. I have friends who are psychiatrists who didn't go through analytic training and you know they have an appreciation but that's because they're them [people who have been through analysis or have other exposure to their field]. But you know I think there are a lot of psychiatrists now who work in a very narrow niche, and in fact their practice is much more narrow than a good analyst who has to think about psychodynamics, and to some extent medication, and to some extent practical matters of everyday living.

In describing the "narrow" practices of nonanalysts, Dr. Ferris sets herself apart from other psychiatrists, whom she and her fellow analysts often describe as less thoughtful, less insightful, and less attuned to patients' needs.

In mainstream psychiatry, being good at DSM diagnosis is an important marker of mastery for clinicians, and the categories have more utility since a practice that is largely psychopharmacological requires very careful diagnosis of symptoms. Furthermore, it ties practitioners to the biomedical model, which connotes rigor. But for most psychoanalysts it is quite the opposite. Prestige is autonomy from the DSM, even as they acknowledge its crucial role, and is likely one of the reasons the Biodynamic and Psychodynamic practitioners talked about diagnosis, instead, as a process of evaluating much more than symptomatology.

Training and the Meaning of Diagnosis

Perhaps one of the clearest distinctions in thinking about DSM diagnosis is how practitioners who are analytically trained (the Biodynamic and Psychodynamic) and those who are not (Biomedical) describe the inclusion of what were once called neuroses and personality disorders in the DSM. When I asked Dr. Park (Biodynamic) whether there was anything in DSM-IV that ideally she would see changed in DSM-5, she told me, "I think they oughta keep their grubby hands off all the important stuff and stick with what they do well. You know, I could answer just the opposite and say they left out neurosis,[4] they should get back to that, but I actually think DSM is very valuable and it should stick to what it's good at, and they should get rid of posttraumatic stress syndrome and dissociation and leave that to us people." As her voice trailed off, Dr. Park finished her thought through subtle, but clearly sarcastic laughter: "Never, never happen, right?" In fact, the DSM-5 did away with the distinction between Axis I (mood disorders) and Axis II (personality) disorders, thereby removing one of the only remaining distinctions between the kinds of illnesses psychoanalysts historically treated (Axis II) and those thought to be more under the purview of Biomedical Psychiatry (Axis I). The "they" in Dr. Park's response refers to the psychiatrists in the DSM working groups who were, at the time of our interview, convening to suggest which diagnoses would be in DSM-5 and how they would be organized.

Dr. Stanley (Biomedical), who described a significant exposure to the psychodynamic model in her training, explains the way DSM categories and insurance coverage converge to cause problems in her practice. She referenced the problem that insurance companies will cover only what is in the DSM and she sighed heavily with a look of exasperation on her face when she described the difficult choices practitioners can face in trying to help their patients afford treatment:

> To be honest, I don't find the DSM very useful. . . . It's not useful in terms of personality disorders. What about these patients that have treatment resistant depression? They have taken out depressive personality disorder, and I have a lot of patients that just sort of live in a depressed

state, where three different medications don't help because they have a depressive temperament that is serving them in some way through a characterologic perspective that is not reflected in DSM-IV at all. And so, when the insurance company calls me up and says why isn't she getting better and I have no language to explain why she is not getting better because the DSM-IV has taken these character pathologies out, which can be incredibly impairing and cause the Axis I to look very treatment resistant.

I asked her what she does in that case or how she responds to the insurance company: "I say she is severely character disordered, that is interfering with her Axis I, and causing her to be treatment resistant, so they either deny me, or you know you do whatever you can to get coverage. But I think that is probably the biggest problem, how do you treat these patients that have severe character pathology that has been taken out of the DSM and how do you justify them not getting better to insurance companies?" Dr. Stanley struggles to properly diagnose and treat her patients, while also making sure that insurance companies will fund those treatments.

On the opposite side of the spectrum is Dr. Clarendon's (Biomedical) statement about one of the ways in which she finds the DSM useful:

> It's extremely well written and its summaries, of course, prognosis, etiological factors, extremely, extremely useful. It's useful with patients. There are many times when I am making a diagnosis, especially a personality disorder and I think, does someone have borderline personality disorder or whether there are different ideas of what that whole thing is about. I will say to the patient let me read you these criteria out of the DSM. Do you think that this fits? And many times patients will say yes that's exactly me, or they will say absolutely not, that's not me. That's helpful to me. Yes, I think those are definite positives.

Despite recognizing problems with the DSM, Dr. Clarendon finds the personality disorder descriptions helpful—the precise diagnoses that psychoanalysts firmly believe should be under their purview and critique as poorly explained in the DSM. From a psychoanalytic perspective, lumping personality disorders in with Axis I conditions is an attempt to make that which is most connected to experience and trauma into something relevant for medical treatment. For a Biomedical Psychiatrist, who does not have the far-ranging training in personality, it's helpful to have descriptions of these disorders and diagnostic categories to guide their treatment.

Though the majority of the practitioners I interviewed, regardless of their training, agreed that they use the DSM for practical purposes, the thinking about the role of diagnosis and the centrality of the DSM varies quite dramatically, especially between the more Biomedical Psychiatrists and the purely Psychodynamic Psychologists. For those with training in psychoanalysis, the DSM may help organize thinking or may simply be used for insurance purposes, but it does not dictate treatment and is only one piece of diagnosis. It is generally a starting point. Dr. Carroll (Biodynamic) explains, "I refer to DSM fairly often if I have to make a formal diagnosis for insurance purposes and that kind of thing . . . but I only resort to them [DSM categories] on occasion. I form a dynamic impression, a diagnostic impression. But I don't ignore symptoms. . . . I'm interested in how they manage their self-esteem, in their personal relationships, to their career, how they might sabotage themselves or stumble over their own feet, their family relationships, their early life, influential developmental figures in their lives." She and I concurred that this sounds very different from a standard DSM diagnosis, which would assess symptom severity and duration, often largely outside the patient's life context. Dr. Carroll wanted it to be clear that she doesn't ignore DSM symptoms but that she is concerned with something deeper. When I asked Dr. Brighton (Psychodynamic) what she takes into account in making a diagnosis, she offered the quintessential explanation for the Psychodynamic group:

> Quality of their affect. Quality of their relationships. Symptoms. What are the symptoms? And the history of the symptoms. Certainly their history, the history of their relationships. I may have said that already, but the history and the quality of their relationships are very central in the diagnosis of their character, if that's what's called for. And the quality of their emotional life. . . . The symptoms really will determine if it's Axis I or Axis II. . . . So Axis II I'm looking at quality of relationships over time and Axis I I'm looking more at the symptoms of anxiety, depression, mood.

Not only did Dr. Brighton point out the importance of assessing the complexity of the patient well beyond symptomatology, but she also makes an important distinction in terms of the relevance of the DSM for different kinds of conditions. The role of DSM in diagnosis depends on whether patients have symptoms of a mood disorder or troubles more directly related to their character and personality. Because psychologists are trained to think about the dynamic, complex elements of character, the DSM is just one element of how they assess patients.

On the other hand, for the most strictly biomedical, such as Dr. Evans, whose practice largely involves treating children with medication, DSM is the central diagnostic tool. When I asked her what role the DSM plays in her practice, she replied, "I go through questionnaires based on DSM. You know there's a rating scale or a diagnostic questionnaire that I go through . . . which is based off the DSM. Because it's structured off the DSM I'm gonna have to say it plays a big role. DSM, it's still the basis in terms of diagnostic symptoms—part of diagnostic evaluation." For Dr. Evans, the central goal is to find the right diagnosis and match the patient with a medication, so patients' interpretations of their symptoms and the larger context of their lives are often much less relevant. In response to my question about why some people regard DSM as the bible of psychiatry, Dr. Butler (Psychodynamic) suggested a key difference in thinking about the DSM between her colleagues who are trained in psychoanalysis and those who are not: "I mean it's a kind of lingua franca, it's just a convenience really. And the psychiatrists I know who are analysts I think don't regard it as that in that biblical fashion. I think they're more sophisticated than that. I mean, maybe psychiatrists who are more biological than that might see it that way." Indeed, most of the Biomedical Psychiatrists do use the DSM in daily practice and think much more categorically than the Biodynamic and Psychodynamic practitioners.

Even the Biomedical Psychiatrists who told me they had some psychodynamic training, while they tended to be a bit more discerning, more like their Biodynamic colleagues, still relied on a formal DSM diagnosis. When I asked her what kind of psychiatry she practices, Dr. Elm (Biomedical) was clear that she wasn't going to "fit into any of my categories" because she uses "innovative techniques . . . that have to do with mind-body integration," particularly for treating patients who have experienced trauma. She did her residency in the mid-1970s; unsurprisingly, her psychiatry training was somewhat "psychoanalytically oriented." Of her patients, 90 percent take medications, but 75 percent are in talk therapy, and she sees only 25 percent for medications only. Dr. Elm also had significant perspective on the field in part because she was nearly sixty at the time of our interview and partly because she has been exposed to a wide range of paradigms in her time in practice. When it comes to the DSM though, Dr. Elm sounds a lot like the rest of her Biomedical Psychiatrist colleagues: "I do a formal history the way they taught me. I go over everything and I have patients fill out a health screening form, just in case I may forget to ask something. That includes a little family history and what they're presenting symptoms on so I have that on the record too." Dr. Elm's description of what she takes into account in making a diagnosis is of a standard, psychiatric practice in line with the biomedical model; in other words, it is largely an analysis of current symptoms and factors related to heritability.

It was Dr. Brighton (Psychodynamic) who astutely observed the origin of the difference between psychoanalysts', particularly Psychodynamic Psychologists' views of the DSM and those of the Biomedical Psychiatrists. It is about "the difference between the two different types of training."

> One type of training is trying to categorize, coming out of the medical model, what's the illness, what's the disease, what kind of pills are we gonna give them? They have four years of training in those pills. That's heavy-duty training, that's what residency is. Psychologists are coming at it with who is the whole person? You can't quickly categorize that. And you wanna have a dynamic formulation, you wanna have an understanding of how this person has been put together. It's a different orientation. What do I think about it? It's their bible but I think it can be extremely limiting and what I see in teaching psychiatrists who are now psychoanalysts it's very interesting to see them try to get out of their bible.

Dr. Brighton assured me that psychoanalytic training "works very hard" at getting psychiatrists to "get out of their bible" and that psychoanalysts do not see the DSM that way. It is clear that having even some training in talk therapy, specifically psychodynamic psychotherapy, makes Biomedical Psychiatrists more critical of the biomedical model, including but not limited to the diagnostic system. Likewise, being a psychiatrist, whether Biomedical or Biodynamic, indicates a greater likelihood to see the benefit of formal diagnosis compared to the Psychodynamic Psychologists.

Perhaps the clearest example of the impact of training and mentorship on practice was my conversation with Dr. Stanley. A Biomedical Psychiatrist by training and trade, Dr. Stanley described her residency program as "very psychodynamic, but also very psychopharmacological." "A lot of the attendings were much more biologically oriented," she explained, which is why she considers herself well trained in the biomedical model. But she thinks about character and personality in addition to DSM categories because her residency made her feel "very well rounded." She explained that she wishes she was more able to describe her patients in psychodynamic language, but she knows she must use the language of the DSM if her patients have any hope for reimbursement. Given the years Dr. Stanley trained, in the early 2000s, I did not expect her to describe any significant psychotherapy training in her residency, but I was wrong:

> I actually had very good psychotherapy training because at the time the residency director and the chairman . . . they were both analysts, they

were both psychiatrists, but were trained as psychoanalysts. [The chairman], he was my supervisor, so I would meet with him once a week for two years, so I mean, that was the training for psychotherapy, but he was an analyst, so a lot of residency programs, your supervisors are not analysts, they are trained in all different ways, but both the residency director and the chairman, they were both analytically trained, and so that's one of the reasons I picked the program.

While Dr. Stanley's course work mirrored that of her cohort in terms of its focus on diagnosis and medication, which is reflected in her practice, where psychopharmacology is the central treatment modality, her training also instilled a sense of the importance of psychodynamic principles, something she sought out, and something she uses as bedrock principles when thinking about her patients. Of her fifty-eight regular patients, eight are medication only, five are talk therapy only, and the rest are in combination treatments. "Unique," in her words, for a Biomedical Psychiatrist, she sees the majority of her patients weekly and even has a couple of patients whom she describes as her most "fragile," whom she sees more than once a week. She describes her approach to treatment with most patients as psychodynamic, and she treats a number of patients who have been diagnosed with borderline personality disorder, a diagnosis squarely in the wheelhouse of psychoanalysts, one practitioners told me is rarely helped with medications alone. When I asked her about deficits in psychiatry today, she told me that there's a lack of training in "how to deal with attachment trauma and insecure attachment styles," which she says can be "incredibly impairing and create a lot of pain." She is troubled that psychiatrists "don't know how to deal with that." In other words, her training in psychodynamic principles, despite her extensive and thorough training in biomedical psychiatry, had a significant impact on the kind of patients she treats and how she thinks about their troubles. Although she doesn't see patients multiple times per week, she employs psychodynamic principles when working with people she thinks will benefit from the approach and is critical of both the rigidity of DSM categorization and the overuse of medication. Dr. Stanley fits the mold of a Biomedical Psychiatrists in many ways and yet, when it comes to diagnosis, she's open to broader issues of personhood and life context because of what she considers an auspicious exposure to psychodynamic ideas.

The Weight of the DSM

Because of the wide-ranging critique of DSM diagnosis within the mental health professions, from social scientists, and even journalists, the DSM has taken on a somewhat larger-than-life role—it is both a tool of practice and a symbolic representation of rigid categorization. As such, the most common gut reaction to my questions about the DSM was often some form of laughter or more overt joking. Practitioners consistently chuckled at my question about the use of the DSM in practice, but they also spoke with concern—even anxiety—about the ubiquity of categorical thinking in mental health treatment and specifically in psychiatry training.

The DSM is indeed one of the main modes by which mental health practice remains squarely within the biomedical model (Horwitz 2002a; Schnittker 2017; Timmermans and Berg 2003a). By using the DSM and thinking in terms of standard diagnostic categories, psychiatrists in particular reinforce the notion that their patients' symptoms are disorders in need of medical treatment. Practitioners point to the DSM's utility in classifying and codifying what are sometimes murky, even ephemeral symptoms. The DSM assists in what Gerrity et al. (1992, 1029) refer to as the "the denial of uncertainty," the main function of which is that it "allows physicians to make potentially threatening situations more understandable and controllable, thus enabling action to take place." Particularly for residents, the DSM is an important organizing structure. And categorization allows for a language with which doctors can communicate and understand one another. As Timmermans and Berg (2003a, 19) suggest, there are two sides to the debate over evidence-based practices: "Because evidence-based medicine integrates clinical acumen with current best evidence, it makes the competent clinician even more competent and less likely to become blinded by experience or theorizing. . . . Critics, on the other hand, charge that evidence-based health care turns clinical practice into bland and unsavory 'cookbook' medicine." My interviewees used this very language—consulting DSM is like following a recipe; it affords predictability but also fosters a lack of creativity.

At the same time as the DSM is useful and necessary in a world dominated by managed care, my interviewees are critical of the diagnostic model. As a representation, even a symbol of the biomedical model of mental illness, our conversations about the DSM necessarily led to discussions of the troubles with modern medicine more generally. The practitioners I spoke with were clear that the DSM promotes what Kleinman (1988) points to as a lack of attention to "illness experience" in modern medicine, or what Mishler (1984) refers to as the patient's "lifeworld," which is largely peripheral, even absent from the DSM model. In training to see patients in terms of diagnostic categories, doctors are focused on finding disorder rather than the deeper meaning of symptoms, as Cassell (2004) notes when he describes medical practice as no longer interested in the stories behind illness or the complete picture of conditions.

My interviewees' descriptions of their use of DSM diagnosis are likewise reminiscent of Luhrmann's (2001, 36) description of residents who are taught to
identify their patients the way one might distinguish between breeds of dogs.
In this way, the use of the DSM epitomizes the empiricism of evidence-based
medicine, and given its centrality to both training and practice, both are sites
of medicalization.

The DSM also allows doctors to take action and to feel connected to biomedicine. Luhrmann (2001, 99) explains, "Biomedical psychiatry is about doing
something, about acting and intervening, the way doctors are supposed to do . . .
the biomedical approach becomes a way to cling to one's doctorly identity."
Some of the Biodynamic Psychiatrists (and one of the Biomedical Psychiatrists)
became irritated with me when they felt I insinuated that psychiatry is in any
way different from other medical fields. For example, while I asked all my
interviewees what major contributions their field has made to society, only the
psychiatrists took this as a slight and in one case even asked me if I would ask
that question of an internist or other medical practitioner. The perceived insin-
uation that I didn't think of their field as being as valid as another medical
discipline alerted me to the importance for at least some of the psychiatrists I
interviewed of maintaining their sense of connection to the field of medicine.

Regardless of how practitioners talk about the DSM, and how they feel about
the manual, it plays at least a meaningful role in each of my interviewee's practices. It plays a more central role in the practice of medical professionals in large
part because there is a connection between a DSM diagnosis and the use of psychotropic medications and in part because all psychiatrists today are trained
extensively in the DSM model of diagnosis (much more so than psychologists).
Younger practitioners learned it in medical school, and even more senior practitioners, who came of professional age before 1980, are required to know the
DSM for licensing exams. Furthermore, the DSM carries the weight of the profession on its shoulders; the widespread use of discrete diagnosis maintains the
sense that the mental health fields (psychiatry in particular) are scientific (Hale
1995; Horwitz 2002a; Schnittker 2017). The DSM serves in the performance of
what Gieryn (1983) calls *boundary work*, separating biomedical psychiatry from
softer, less scientific forms of practice and demarcating it as a medical field. In
codifying the kinds of conditions deemed appropriate to treat and those in need
of treatment, the DSM situates both patients' troubles and practitioners themselves in the biomedical model; it anchors psychiatrists to the technology of
their field and allows them to identify with the larger profession of medicine
(Horwitz 2002a; Schnittker 2017).

Psychoanalysts, because of their training in psychodynamic theory and talk therapy, are generally more critical of the manual and recognize the DSM as a text that tries to do too much. For the Psychodynamic Psychologists, the DSM is sometimes useful in a basic way for organizing their thinking, and it must be used for insurance purposes, but they describe it much more as an a priori set of standards to which the field, and therefore they, conforms, rather than a process they are a part of. In fact, for psychoanalytically trained doctors, the rigidity of the DSM pushes them to be more discerning and prevents them from following DSM as doctrine. In this way, many of the Psychodynamic and the Biodynamic doctors regard themselves as deeper thinkers and even more expert than their Biomedical counterparts. The Biodynamic Psychiatrists in particular, because of their dual training, often indicated that shrewd use of the DSM provides a sense of prestige—a sort of antidote to the rigidity of the categories. My interviewees were clear on the importance of "good clinical judgment," which Luhrmann (2001) describes as a common marker for residents in becoming respectable doctors. Yet, particularly for the psychoanalysts, being discerning and not using the DSM in a literal manner figures prominently in their sense of being a sophisticated practitioner. Many of my interviewees reported that they are careful not to be overly categorical in their thinking about people, who, almost all of them remind me, do not fit neatly into diagnostic categories. As Whooley (2010, 466) reminds us, "The use of the DSM is varied, representing a complex negotiation between individual psychiatrists' views of mental illness, various constraints placed on their autonomy by outside actors and the local exigencies of the clinical interaction." My interviewees' fear, of course, is that many practitioners, particularly those in the early stages of their career, are not judicious.

At the same time, the Biodynamic Psychiatrists particularly tend to underestimate the tacit role the DSM plays in practice. Although most of them don't use standard checklists, they are still influenced by diagnostic thinking. As Dr. Warren explained, when she is thinking about diagnoses, she may not be directly referring to DSM, but those DSM categories that she learned in medical school and used in her residency all the time are there in her mind. They have become a major, if not the predominant, way of making sense of patients' symptoms. Bowker and Star (2000, 287) remind us, "Categories are historically situated artifacts and, like all artifacts, are learned as part of membership in communities of practice." Light (1980, 160) describes the internalization of diagnostic categories as a major feature of psychiatry training: "Learning how to diagnose is a skill which psychiatric residents must learn before all others. . . .

Paradoxically, however, as residents become more seasoned practitioners, diagnosis no longer retains this preeminent role; one learns to formulate a plan of treatment more by feel and common sense. But this may be no paradox at all if 'feel and common sense' have by that time become imbued with the psychiatric mode of diagnosis." The diagnostic categories are so much a part of the psychiatric worldview that practitioners leave their residency feeling as though they are classifying natural, objectively observable phenomena. Despite its relatively straightforward role in practice and practitioners' recognition that the DSM creates potentially dangerous outcomes for both clinicians and patients, it is more than a textbook; for psychiatrists in particular, the DSM is a cognitive framework for assessment. Schnittker (2017, 112) argues that clinicians have more discretion than researchers in terms of how they use the DSM because "the work of clinicians prevents them from thinking about diagnosis in the pure way envisioned by the DSM." This is true; the patient sitting in front of the practitioner is rarely seen simply as the features of their diagnosis. At the same time, my interviewees described a range of ways in which DSM thinking circumscribes their thinking and practice. And most are concerned about the rigid thinking DSM diagnosis encourages in junior practitioners.

For the practitioners who are the most wedded to the psychoanalytic model, particularly the more senior psychoanalysts, the DSM also symbolizes the relegation of the psychodynamic model to second-class citizenship in the field. Even the most psychodynamically oriented practitioners recognize the need for standardization, as is clear in one of the central selling points of the DSM: the promise of scientificity in the form of an evidence-based model—precisely what critics of psychoanalysis think it lacks. Practitioners' attitudes about etiology and diagnosis are connected to their training and credentials, which also impact what their practice looks like—whether they prescribe medications, what role they think medications play in practice, and whether they see talk therapy as a useful mode of treatment. Especially to senior practitioners, particularly psychoanalysts, any conversation about the DSM is intrinsically rooted in debates around the role of talk therapy and medication in treatment. It is to these issues that I turn in chapter 4.

Etiological Considerations and the Tools of the Trade

The Role of Medication and Talk Therapy in Practice

Dr. Troy, a Biomedical Psychiatrist, is heavily involved in training psychiatry residents in one of New York's prominent hospitals. Her teaching and mentoring role afforded her an ability to clearly articulate what are more implicit notions for many of her colleagues. Especially when I asked her about etiology, she captured the essence of what I'd heard from many of her colleagues. "The best way to think about many of the illnesses that we have," she told me, "is that there is a combination of vulnerability and insult, and you have got to have both. One isn't enough. You have to have vulnerability, susceptibility and you have to receive one, two, three, sometimes more noxious stimuli." The development of mental health troubles involves vulnerability. What that susceptibility entails is not always clear, however, and practitioners have a range of ideas about its etiology and how best to manage its outcomes.

When I asked Dr. Troy what the dominant paradigm is in psychiatry today, she was quick to tell me it's "prescribing," which she reported "with sadness" because even though she is a Biomedical Psychiatrist, her residency program was run by psychiatrists with allegiances to the psychodynamic model, which she finds helpful. When we discussed what she thinks the dominant paradigm ought to be for understanding psychiatric illness, she told me it's "hard to answer," which became clear as she described the complexity and even ambiguity around etiology, diagnosis, and treatment. When I inquired about etiology, Dr. Troy was clear that she divides her patients into categories based on her assessment of whether they have a "physiological aberration."

Sometimes it is an illness just like an illness in physical medicine that is a disturbance in physiology that leads to various symptoms. There, the paradigm can be the same as in medicine—let's find a link 'cause if we can, until we find the cause let's treat the symptoms, let's do what makes the symptoms better. So, we don't know how, we don't have antibiotics yet, but we do know if we give you Tylenol your fever goes down, so let's give you Tylenol. That's fine. But that's only one slice of the illness of all psychiatric disturbances that we see.

The other part is ineffective coping, not necessarily because of physiological aberration or because of some sort of chemical imbalance so to speak, but because the coping skills weren't acquired. Or the compensatory mechanism, to make it even broader, for that disturbance weren't acquired. I mean we all face mental disturbances, we all face disturbances of all kinds, and we all compensate for them in different ways. For those of us that learn to compensate is to go out to a bar and get slammed do that, and then all those people because of biology some people end up getting addicted, but they wouldn't have gotten addicted if they hadn't had the combination of the bad wiring *and* this bad learning. So, I think that if you have a slice of people who have not the bad wiring but only the improper learning or the inadequate learning, so there is a solution for that, but it isn't necessarily a pharmaceutical solution, and I think we recognize that. . . .

And then the third slice of patients fit into neither of those categories and it is hard to sort of qualify them. Folks who have acquired skills, they don't really have any clear physiological aberrations, at least that we can tell right now, but for a variety of reasons they're—and I am going to use the biological paradigm, I mean, in the end it's all biological paradigm, it's all controlled by our brains—there's a disruption in the normal equilibrium of brain function. Sometimes it's the part of the brain that is responsible for our sense of self and when that disruption occurs because of whatever is going on around us that leads to what looks like an illness, but then the treatment for that may just be—I am going to go out on a limb here and use not a good phrase—but the treatment may just be hand holding, or the "this too shall pass" thing, and often it does. But we have arrived at a time where that becomes very quickly labeled as an illness because outwardly it looks like one. I mean a great example of that is someone who is reeling after the death of someone that is close to them, and you know we would all say for the first month, well you know their spouse just died, you know it's understandable. But then two months later we would say it's not understandable. But who should say it's two months? Do I get to decide it's two months? Maybe it's two months to me, but maybe three months for you? But does that mean that you have an illness and I don't or that the next person who for whom it lasts six months? So, I think that that's the third set of people. That it's a disequilibrium that is temporary that gets labeled, which is why I think that whatever symptoms one presents with, it is essential that we place it against the backdrop of their lives and that we don't just view them in isolation. Because once you have the person's life on the canvas and you place the symptoms upon that canvas, whatever color or texture that canvas has, then you can decide is this a physiological aberration or is it an improperly or inadequately acquired compensatory skill set? Or is it this temporary disturbance that is not aberrant necessarily but a variant? It's a variant.

Dr. Troy separates patients into three categories, each with treatment implications. The first are patients who, she explains, have a true illness. They are the best candidates for medication; their symptoms are comparable to a fever, which can be alleviated with Tylenol. Like with a pathogen, she assumes some sort of biological vulnerability causes these disorders. The patients in the second group do not have what she calls "bad wiring," but instead did not learn to cope well enough with life's troubles; their vulnerability is psychological and a deficit in learning. These patients may not necessarily need medication, though she would likely recommend treatment of some kind. Dr. Troy suggests that there can be a combination of problematic coping and "bad wiring" as in addiction, where someone might compensate for lack of appropriate coping skills by using substances. But becoming addicted to those substances, Dr. Troy suggests, is attributable to something more innate than managing emotions or learning. Finally, Dr. Troy describes a group of patients whose troubles do not seem to indicate any clear illness, but who she believes have some kind of disruption in their sense of self, although she sees these troubles as being rooted in the brain as well. While she is concerned about overdiagnosis because she says this last group often looks like they have an illness when they may not, Dr. Troy was clear that "it's all controlled by their brains." Even though she sees all symptoms, whether they are a disruption in the sense of self or intense sadness as rooted in biology, she does not see them all as illness. How Dr. Troy and other practitioners puzzle out the type of vulnerability they believe their patients have dictates their treatment decisions.

Dr. Troy drew connections between assessments of etiology, diagnosis, and treatment. In her description of trying to parse out whether a patient has a "disturbance in physiology" is an evaluation of whether a patient needs medication. Dr. Troy's explanation of etiology lays out what most of the psychiatrists I interviewed call the biopsychosocial model. When I asked about the causes of the problems their patients bring to treatment, both the Biodynamic and Biomedical Psychiatrists often told me their answer would be "boring" or "not that different" from what others had told me, which was true—the description of etiology as biopsychosocial is textbook, straight from their medical training. Because of her psychodynamically trained mentors, Dr. Troy had a sense that social norms, context, and personal experience drive symptoms and diagnosis, but she privileged biology over other factors, as did most Biomedical and Biodynamic Psychiatrists. Psychodynamic Psychologists also alluded to biological, psychological, and social sources of the troubles they treat, though they did not use the term "biopsychosocial" and generally privileged the psychological. In their attempts to make sense of their patients' wide range of symptoms and experiences, practitioners rely on their ideas about etiology and the tools of their trade—medication and various forms of talk therapy.

Etiology: "A Combination of Vulnerability and Insult"

Dr. Troy laid out the ideal sources she thinks practitioners ought to consider when they think about etiology—biology, psychology, and environment. Vulnerability in any of these areas, she explained, can lead to illness. Though her colleagues agree that it is important to consider all sources, the majority of the Biomedical Psychiatrists I spoke with overwhelmingly privilege biological factors. Consider Dr. Doughty's (Biomedical) ideas about etiology:

> I actually think of it as sort of, for most of the stuff that I treat generally, not the schizophrenia, not for stuff that is really clearly just biologically orientated, but the depressive disorders and the anxiety disorders, the way I think about it is that you are sort of born with a biological predilection, which kind of sets a threshold. Then what acts on that threshold are sort of your environmental stresses and the coping skills that you have developed to deal with them. So, I think that there are some people that have very low thresholds and it takes very little to push them into some sort of illness. And, you meet people like that. People who—everyone does—people who seem like they cannot deal and maybe some people think of them as having characterological weakness, but maybe what they really have is just a very low threshold, and it doesn't take them very much to tip them over into an episode. . . . I think that if you experience a little bit of pain, a vaccination kind of, an immunization, you kind of

develop coping skills for cognitively understanding that it is part of life, and then also for dealing with adversity when it comes up. So, those three things interact. Even if you have a really low threshold if your life goes swimmingly well and you don't hit any major snags then maybe you will never have an episode. So, I think of it as sort of, in my head three different factors that sort of interact with each other.

Like Dr. Troy, Dr. Doughty is one of the Biomedical Psychiatrists who trained in the 1980s in a residency program that was still dominated by psychodynamic thinking. But she informed me that her hospital began to "move into a more biological paradigm" when she was there. As such, she thinks about character and environment, but overwhelmingly feels like there is a biological mechanism underlying the development of symptoms, setting what she describes as a "threshold." Citing remarkably similar etiological factors, Dr. Brooks (Biomedical) told me,

> Well, I think there's some biological loading, probably genetic in large part. And the environmental—I think social interactions and issues contribute. There are other biological things out there. I mean toxins and this and that and you know someone has a tumor in their brain or something so there are those things as well, so it depends on the disorder. You know, schizophrenia is probably the result of many different biological things and the brain's too complicated, we don't understand it yet. Looking for a genetic cause, the age of the father, whatever. You know it could be all those. I mean it's hard to say. I don't think we have it yet.

Though most list what they think are key causes, they are aware their notions of etiology involve a great deal of speculation without concrete evidence, a problem for psychiatry.

The Biodynamic Psychiatrists are often analogous to their Biomedical counterparts in their thinking about etiology, but many, like Dr. Dean (Biodynamic), emphasize additional factors beyond inherited vulnerability that they see as implicated in the development of distress:

> Well, it's always a combination of factors. Someone has a psychiatric illness, okay, it's for a number of reasons. Firstly, because they had some kind of inborn genetic vulnerability or biological, they were born with a vulnerability, and upon that vulnerability was played some stress perhaps in interaction with the parent. A parent who might have gotten away fine with a child who wasn't vulnerable, but this interaction brings about some kind of a deficit of some sort so it's not nature versus nurture, it's

nature and nurture interacting together always. . . . Someone may have a trauma, that's more unusual—but if someone's been in a war for example. Everyone has their breaking point, ya know.

In Dr. Dean's description of an "inborn genetic vulnerability" is the centrality of biomedical thinking and the clear assumption that biology is in constant interplay with "nurture," in this case represented by parenting and war. Dr. Ferris (Biodynamic) explains her similar philosophy on etiology:

> Well, first you start with genes. . . . Then, under certain circumstances, growing up in certain families or being exposed to traumatic experiences or growing up in a family with parents or siblings who can tolerate more things and contain it, someone would be more or less vulnerable if they have the genes. . . . And you know maybe some people, if they grow up with enough resourcefulness can kind of counterbalance what may sway another person into becoming deeply depressed about something. But I think . . . so much of it is just in the genes and the chromosomes.

Though environment (nurture) is important, it is rarely assigned primacy the way nature (as genetics) is. In Dr. Ferris's description is also an emphasis on overcoming the environment, but an almost inevitability about genetic factors. The same sentiment is clear in Dr. Warren's (Biodynamic) description of etiology for her child and adolescent patients: "There's a huge genetic component to a lot of things. I would say that's a very important part. . . . Obviously environmental components play a role, it's not that I don't think they do and certain kids have had more traumas and more parental deprivation and more inconsistent parenting and all of that plays a big role, but I certainly think that a kid's either genetic endowment or the way they come into this world plays a huge role too." There is a general sentiment that "how people come into the world" is responsible for either normal or pathological functioning in early and later life. Biodynamic Psychiatrists described a sense of well preparedness for treating patients precisely because they can draw from both psychopharmacology and psychodynamic psychotherapy. The Biodynamic Psychiatrists feel they (and their patients) benefit from the multiplicative effect of using both biomedical and dynamic treatments together, which is clear in their descriptions of having more treatment tools than their Biomedical and Psychodynamic counterparts.

While the Psychodynamic Psychologists also believe biology is implicated in mental health troubles, their notion of vulnerability is quite different. Dr. Butler (Psychodynamic) explains the widely accepted notion of the interplay between biology and environment:

[Symptoms] can be genetically-based in part, and they can also be experientially based, and they arrive and there's a kind of diathesis model where you may inherit genetic vulnerabilities, but it may take adverse environmental conditions to bring it out. And I do think family dynamics can be—heaven knows we're all exposed to them in one way or another—but I think people essentially get programmed with a whole lot of default assumptions and expectations and behaviors growing up that in a sense you could see therapy as a way of reprogramming almost.

Like Dr. Troy, Dr. Butler, in explaining etiology, also describes her conceptualizations about treatment. She explains that genetic vulnerabilities are triggered by environmental conditions—but what is "programmed," in her words, is tied to socialization and thus can be reprogrammed or perhaps even deprogrammed. Though she starts out with genetics, her emphasis is on learned assumptions and behavior. Psychodynamic Psychologists tended to assume that there are somewhat unclear biological derivations of mental health troubles, but they are not the focus of treatment, and they spend little time discussing vulnerability as an innate quality. Dr. Kane (Psychodynamic) described the etiology of psychiatric troubles as a combination of "nature and nurture. Biology and environment." She explained, "I think more about the environmental, more about human nature, but I'm aware that biology contributes." Dr. Haman (Psychodynamic) likewise told me, "I'm always thinking, or often I guess, about a patient's early life. . . . I think with some patients who are more likely to be the patients taking medications, I also think about biological factors. . . . I don't really think about the biological much with the other patients, I think it's not really fair to say I think much at all about that." If a patient is taking a medication, it might push a Psychodynamic Psychologist to think more about biology, particularly if a medication seems to be helpful, but biological factors were rarely their central concern, and they never described their perspective on etiology simply as "biopsychosocial" in the way that Biodynamic Psychiatrists are taught it. Further, while the Biodynamic Psychiatrists always reminded me that I would likely hear the same answer from their colleagues (and indeed I did), the psychodynamic group gave much more detailed and varied answers, especially about what the "psycho" actually entails.

Yet even the Psychodynamic Psychologists, who are presumably the least medically oriented, were sometimes quick to point out the influence of biology, especially for patients with severe symptoms. Like Dr. Haman, who thinks more about biology when a patient takes medication, Dr. Butler (Psychodynamic) explains that though it's often hard to tell which patients will benefit from which kind of treatment, the more serious the condition, the more likely she is to refer someone for a medication consultation, and the more likely she is to attribute symptoms to biology:

> In a sense, everything is biological. We're biological organisms, but for some people even if they come in depressed, the very fact of being in treatment will lift them out of it. But for someone who has a really sort of unshakable, gloomy, deep-seeded depression that doesn't really respond to psychological, therapeutic interventions, then I would definitely think about it [medication]. And you know it's often the case with eating disorders that an antidepressant can really help a patient sort of get to a place where they can better deal with the problem. And anyone who's bipolar or has a history of bipolar I would certainly refer. . . . If you can resolve some of that really serious symptomatology, then it makes the patient much more able to cope, to function, to engage in the therapy in fact. I see it as putting them on a somewhat more normal plateau as it were, where they're not so constantly overwhelmed by fighting depression or anxiety that they can't really do much else.

In one way, Dr. Butler sounds a lot like a psychiatrist when she says "everything is biological," but her tone was somewhat mocking—as if to say, "biology is everything and it's nothing." Despite her sarcasm, it was clear she feels medicine is warranted when patients present with serious symptomatology.

Practitioners in all three groups describe the influence of biology, psychology, and the social environment as important factors in the development of mental health troubles. A notion of vulnerability is central to the descriptions of etiology for all three types of practitioners. However, both Biomedical and Biodynamic Psychiatrists tended to privilege biological, heritable vulnerability, while the Psychodynamic Psychologists tend to focus primarily on psychological and environmental factors in creating a vulnerability to experience mental health troubles, and thought more about biology only when patients have very severe symptoms, which usually involve psychopharmacological intervention. As Dr. Lewis (Biodynamic) decries of the biopsychosocial model, "What every training program [in psychiatry] will tell you . . . if you were to learn psychiatry . . . that's what people think that they are going to get. Ya know, it's really not." Dr. Lewis was clear that in psychiatry training there is a significant emphasis on the biomedical model, which goes hand in hand with the extensive training in DSM diagnosis. The result is that most of the psychiatrists I spoke with (with the exception of those who trained before 1980) told me that etiology is biopsychosocial, yet when we really started talking about their patients and their practice, it was clear that biology tends to outweigh the psycho and social. Furthermore, the "social" does not generally extend beyond proximate environment (often described as immediate family). Psychodynamic Psychologists are perhaps more genuinely biopsychosocial in their thinking, even though they're not taught it as such; they consider the roles of relationships, culture, and social forces in ways I did not hear as often from other practitioners.

Practitioners' ideas about which patients need medication and which patients can benefit from talk therapy alone are grounded in ideas about etiology. The belief that medications work relies on the belief that symptoms arise from the biological mechanisms medications are meant to target, which is perhaps most clear in Dr. Carroll's (Biodynamic) description of major changes she's seen in treatment since she trained in psychiatry. When she trained, she explained, "there was no psychopharmacology . . . just some heavy tranquilizers and they were experimenting with antidepressants. Originally, I did psychotherapy with people who would go into these depressions, and of course, when they're in major depression, their thoughts are repetitive and we just used to sweat it out. Finally, the depression would lift spontaneously, and we had the illusion that we helped them work out of the depression, when it really is a biological illness, in most cases." Dr. Carroll describes not only the connection between the use of medication and the belief in biological etiology, but also that medications offered a tool for treating debilitating symptoms that practitioners had struggled to treat with psychodynamic psychotherapy alone. Psychologists describe some underlying biology as one of the reasons for referring patients to psychopharmacology consultations. Yet to engage in long-term talk therapy, practitioners need to believe their patients can talk through their troubles—that the conditions they treat are not entirely coded in genetics—or there would be little purpose to this kind of work.

Medication

People Deserve Symptom Relief: Medication for Acuity and Severity

Severity and duration, two key criteria set out in the DSM for diagnosis, figure in all my interviewees' thinking about when to use medication. When I asked for indicators that medication would help a patient, there was a consensus among both psychiatrists and psychologists that they prescribe or refer patients for medication consultations when symptoms interfere with daily functioning; psychopharmacology is for situations where the severity of symptoms is such that a patient's normal life (judged as such by the patient, the doctor, or some combination of the two) is in jeopardy, and when those symptoms have persisted for enough time to warrant intervention. Dr. Nelson's (Biodynamic) response to my question about what role medication plays in her practice was typical: "I see it as the shortest route to alleviate pain—not necessarily suffering, but you know if someone fits into a DSM diagnosis that medicine treats I basically feel like it's my obligation as a physician to offer it up." Dr. Nelson references an earlier conversation about whether she differentiated between pain and suffering. Here, she affirmed her notion that pain is more acute (more of a symptom), while suffering is a more existential state. In doing so, she also established what she thinks the biomedical model is useful for: alleviating pain quickly. In that sense, pain is linked to the biomedical model; it can be treated with psychotropic medications (like Tylenol for a fever as Dr. Troy explained earlier). Suffering is more under the purview of the psychoanalyst. Biomedical Psychiatrists were far less likely to make a distinction between the two.

Dr. Hart (Biomedical) described the overarching explanation for using medicine when she said it "can help provide quick relief for some patients." She continued, "I think it's a very helpful tool in treatment. I think, in the context of a whole treatment, it can provide a lot of relief to people. I think these are biologically-driven conditions in many cases, so I think—the medicines are not perfect by any means—but I think they can correct some imbalances, abnormalities, they can settle down the nervous system at times, and they can offer a tremendous amount." When I asked more specifically what elements of a diagnosis would indicate a need for medication, Dr. Hart explained that what she looks for is evidence of "how acute" a problem is. Severity, which includes how a patient is functioning, and duration, if a problem persists over enough time, mean medication is the best option. Dr. Elm (Biomedical) explained, "If someone comes to me and they are suffering terribly and have been for a while, and they're seeking medication I will be very open to the use of medication very quickly under that circumstance. Even if I think that over time something else might be helpful." Dr. Elm recommends talk therapy in addition to medication, but the goal is first to reduce the severity of the patients' symptoms.

Dr. Brighton (Psychodynamic) also informed me that her decision making about referring patients for medication "has to do with functioning." She explains of her patients that "if their functioning's falling down badly, they're at risk for losing their job, not sleeping, gaining a tremendous amount of weight," she would call on a "medical doctor" for a referral. Dr. Kent (Psychodynamic) describes her threshold for decisions about when to refer patients for medication: "If they're very depressed and they don't seem to be functioning, then I would definitely refer them for medication, or sometimes, if they're having very bad obsessional anxiety or sleep problems." For Psychodynamic Psychologists as well, a certain symptom acuity leads them to refer a patient to a psychiatrist for medication. Dr. Adams (Psychodynamic) explains, "I think some people suffer unnecessarily. I think a certain amount of suffering . . . is part of life and should not be thought of as something to get rid of. But then there's, for example, if somebody is up all night, if somebody is really not sleeping, you know, they shouldn't have to deal with that. Or, if somebody is plagued with suicidal thoughts all the time. Or, somebody might really commit suicide. . . . Or somebody is just agitated all the time." Though there is normal suffering (described by other interviewees as anything from sadness because of the loss of a parent or spouse to anxiety because of a serious illness like cancer), Dr. Adams explains that there is also a point at which suffering is too much to bear for a patient; practitioners are on the lookout for whether severity is beyond what is tolerable for both the patient and the practitioner. This is often what interviewees describe as the driving force for patients to enter into treatment in the first place. For instance, Dr. Kent (Psychodynamic) explained that patients tend to come see her when "they just feel terrible and don't know what else to do. In one of a variety of ways—they're depressed or something bad has happened to them." While pain and suffering may lead patients to treatment, if their symptoms are too intense, medications are often a first step, and talk therapy might follow later, or in some cases, they might begin simultaneously.

Recall Dr. Sutter's (Biomedical) description of the three categories she divides her patients into (chapter 2), an explanation for how she thinks about using medications:

> I think of the people who, they just need medication. There's no question. And I'll say to them, "I think it would really be a huge mistake for you not to try a medication." Those are the people where they have serious depression or serious anxiety or serious attention deficit disorder or some bipolar disorder or psychosis—things that medications work really well for. It's just stupid not to take them. So, it's like having high blood pressure. You wouldn't go into a doctor's office and say, "I'm gonna talk to you about your high blood pressure and try and help mellow you out." You'd say, "Look, you have blood pressure that could really kill you and it's making your life—it's gonna cause all sorts of bad things, so you need medicine." Those people I say, "I really think it would be a huge mistake if you don't take medicine."
>
> Then there's the group of people where I say it's sort of optional, where I think it would help, but they could decide and they have to weigh the pros and cons and the side effects. It's not that medicines are side effect free. And I'll discuss the side effects with them and then I'll say to them,

"You know, you can try and you'll decide if you think it's helping or not." . . . Those are the people who have sort of mild depression or mild anxiety where cognitive behavioral therapy or some sort of therapy can make a big difference in terms of learning various relaxation techniques . . . someone who has panic attacks, someone who has phobia of planes, for instance, you can give them medicine. But also, my office mate . . . does amazing cognitive behavioral therapy with anxiety disorders. I say to them, "There's a treatment. It works really well. It's not drugs. You will get cured and you could do that."

And then there's a third where I just think they don't need medicine. Or they can't be on the medicines. I have one guy who had a heart attack and he really needs medicine for ADHD but he can't be on it. Or I have another guy who had a congenital heart problem and again, he really needed ADHD medicine.

For the second and third groups (and sometimes for the first group as well), Dr. Sutter recommends talk therapy. Although she reports with great specificity that she prescribes medications for 97 percent of her patients, only 25 percent of her practice is made up of patients whom she sees for medication only. This means that a significant number of her patients are in combined treatments, although her brand of talk therapy is more supportive and far less in-depth than is the case for her psychoanalytic counterparts.[1]

While Biomedical Psychiatrists use medications to reduce symptoms, Biodynamic Psychiatrists and Psychodynamic Psychologists are more likely to explain that the purpose of medication is not only to reduce symptoms but to allow patients to further deal with the sources of their problems. Dr. Elliot (Biodynamic) explains that medication is

to relieve symptoms that are troublesome enough to interfere with the person coping with their life. Let's say obsessive thoughts or depression or anxiety. So it can help relieve symptoms. It can reduce symptoms so that the person can then cope better and even work on their underlying problems better. . . . Let's say a person is anxious. You tamp down their anxiety, you have to give them a sleeping pill to get them unanxious or maybe that won't even do it, but there is a level in which something is so unbearable that's all the person can focus on.

While interference with normal or routine functioning and/or the level of suffering reported by the patient are the main indicators for the use of medicines, for psychoanalysts in particular, medicine is often described as a way to get the patient to a point where their symptoms aren't so intense that they cannot even think about the causes of their troubles or make use of in-depth talk therapy.

Medicine as a Catalyst for Talk Therapy

Practitioners describe severe and long-standing symptoms (which both interfere with functioning) as being rooted in biology and neurochemistry. As such, many practitioners explain that medication is the most useful way to treat those symptoms. But particularly those trained in psychoanalysis also describe the utility of medications as an effective way to facilitate successful talk therapy. Dr. Halsey (Biodynamic) confirms that one of the central goals of medication is to "decrease the intensity" of symptoms so that patients are "more willing to think about things, reflect on things, hear what you have to say." Without medications, she says, "if they are so stuck in being upset and angry that they're just overwhelmed you can't do any therapy. So they [talk therapy and medication] do work hand in hand."

There is widespread agreement among my psychoanalyst interviewees that when patients are in pain, their ability to make use of talk therapy is stifled; in order to benefit from any kind of talk therapy, then, medication is beneficial and even necessary. Dr. Madison (Biodynamic) tells me, "People can actually be more thoughtful, more reflective when they're not so miserable." Dr. Brighton (Psychodynamic) likewise explains that medication "can play a very, very beneficial role. . . . Depression lifts, the thinking is so much clearer and the patient can actually tolerate more looking into themselves. . . . So it opens up the thinking and in the opening up of the thinking is typically better capacity to do a good psychotherapy. . . . The less crippled the patient is with the symptoms, the more able they are to look at their overall behavior and the way they're doing in their lives." Insight and deeper analysis of the cause of symptoms, Dr. Brighton explained, aren't possible when someone feels overwhelmed by symptoms or thought styles associated with conditions like depression that, in her words, "cripple" a patient. She explained further, "If their pain is very high and they're into tremendous self-damning, depressive thinking, they actually can't do treatment because every insight leads to what a schmuck I am, ya know. And you have to lift that enough so it opens up the thinking and in the opening up of the thinking is typically better capacity to do a good psychotherapy." Dr. Sullivan (Biodynamic) summarizes the "twofold" purpose of medicine: ". . . to reduce the symptom and then, for example, an anxiety symptom is reduced enough that the patient is calm enough to do dynamic work to get through, for example, a block in being satisfied in a relationship or pursuing more what they want at work." Dr. Clarendon's mentors were psychodynamic psychiatrists, and she was the only Biomedical Psychiatrist to describe medication's role in assisting talk therapy rather than purely for symptom relief. She practices more talk therapy than any other Biomedical Psychiatrist, and she told me,

> As we know from the [clinical trials] of antidepressants that basically a third of the patients respond substantially, and then you know if you go through the other half a dozen treatments the remaining two-thirds don't respond, half of those won't respond and you are left with the unfortunate one-third who don't get much benefit of anything. . . . Medication is, it's not a good bet. It's one amongst many treatments, you know. Patients are coming to me to get medication. It's up to me to try and give them the sense of what they can expect and what they can't expect. I almost always recommend that they have psychotherapy in addition to medication. I think increasingly the feeling is moving to an understanding that medication itself may not be the thing that really produces lasting therapeutic change, but the medication creates an environment or creates—there's a recent article—creates plasticity in the brain that then allows for the therapy or other environmental things to become effective, so you know I talk to patients about how medication is not, so it's one of the things. It's one amongst a number of other treatments.

Despite the Psychodynamic Psychologists' inability to prescribe medication, they too refer patients for psychopharmacology assessments in part because they hope it will facilitate the work they do with their patients.

Since the Biomedical Psychiatrists were more likely to describe the key sources of patients' troubles as biological, it follows that altering neurotransmitters would be the goal of treatment. Furthermore, since the central tool of their treatment is psychopharmacology, they tended to see it as a means to an end rather than a way to facilitate another form of treatment. Psychodynamic and Biodynamic practitioners, by contrast, aim to get at the other sources of illness, and they view medications as a potential tool to allow them to do that.

Concerns about the Appropriate Use of Medications

Aside from the three most biomedical of the psychiatrists whose practices are exclusively psychopharmacological, all my interviewees described some wariness toward the use of medications, a topic of contention particularly for Psychodynamic Practitioners who practice talk therapy exclusively, but who exist in a field dominated by biomedical thinking and practice. Some of the Biodynamic Psychiatrists were also critical of the overuse of medications, as they are keenly aware that the patients they see in long-term talk therapy treatments, who are often taking medications, are not always helped by them, and rarely by psychopharmacology alone. This also confirms for them, the longer they are in practice, that etiology is not just biological. The Psychodynamic Psychologists and older Biodynamic Psychiatrists tended to be the most critical of medication-based treatments (although practitioners in all three groups have concerns). Dr. Kent (Psychodynamic) tells me, "I think it's tragic for many people who are sort of bogged up on medication. I mean, it's bad. It's bad for practice because many people expect to be cured in a quick way." She also notes, "It certainly seems to be bad for training in psychotherapy." In short, my interviewees feel the overuse of medication has deleterious effects on patients and on practitioners. Dr. Kent is careful, however, to add that she is "not at all against medication." In fact, she says, "I'm a big proponent of appropriately used medication." She also says she is "conflicted" about how much of a problem it is that psychiatry is so medicine focused because "it's psychiatry's job to do that." This sentiment is substantiated by several of the Biomedical Psychiatrists who explain that most of their patients come to them specifically because they can prescribe medications, and because they, as psychiatrists, are the only mental health practitioners who can do this. Patients who come into treatment knowing they want medicines are likely to go to someone who can prescribe them. Yet for Psychodynamic Psychologists there is a leeriness toward medications and particularly toward using them alone to treat symptoms.

With the exception of the some of the Biomedical Psychiatrists, the majority of my interviewees were careful to describe themselves as thoughtful about medicines and wanted me to know that they do not see themselves as overly aggressive in their recommendations of medications. The Biomedical Psychiatrists, too, recognize the critique of their field as too dominated by medications as treatment. Dr. Stanley (Biomedical) was clear: "I'm not a real pill pusher. I, only if someone is really, really suffering and I think a medication can help them, but I don't push pills, I refuse to talk to pharmaceutical reps, I won't let them in. I am actually mean to them. So, I only give mediation if I think it will decrease someone's suffering." Though Dr. Stanley doesn't have formal training in psychoanalysis, because her mentors in residency were psychodynamically trained, she too is oriented toward meaning and thinks deeply about patients' experiences; because she thinks about the psychodynamic roots of patients' troubles, she is also more likely to think about treatment as something beyond medication. Dr. Hart (Biomedical), who trained in the 1980s, acknowledged that her residency "evolved" as she was in it. She told me her training "started out being psychodynamic with a lot of emphasis on psychoanalytic teachings from the past, but certainly had a very strong biological piece to it as well." In other words, her mentors were both psychopharmacologists and psychoanalysts. As such, she explained, "psychiatrists do people a tremendous injustice if they're just, 'take Prozac and call me in a week'" (she was equally forthcoming about her feeling that practitioners who treat a highly symptomatic patient without medication are negligent—a critique reminiscent of those levied against psychoanalysis even in its heyday). Her worry about overly rigid treatments may explain why all of her patients are in combined treatments.

Particularly the psychoanalysts reminded me that "medication is an overvalued tool." Furthermore, it was not uncommon, particularly for Biodynamic Psychiatrists, to note that the mechanism responsible for patients' reduced symptomatology is not well understood. Dr. Sterling (Biodynamic) describes these unknowns as one of the exciting things about her field:

> I think that one of the appealing things to me about being a psychiatrist at this point is because so little is understood about etiology and therefore there's a huge amount of discoveries still yet to be made, and a feeling of excitement around trying to understand it. . . . I think whatever understanding we have of etiology is so incredibly far away from the actual complexity of who we are that it almost feels like silly to try and speculate. I mean take the SSRIs for example—that they are *selective* serotonin reuptake inhibitors. I feel like that's about one of maybe a thousand things that they do. Maybe that's the most incidental. I have no idea. Luckily, we did find something that seems to work somewhat, somewhat, you know not incredibly well. But I think a lot of medications in medicine are like that; we have some idea of how they work. I mean some more than others.

Some practitioners presented the unknowns of their field as troubling, while others, like Dr. Sterling, simply think of the field—and particularly medications—as a work in progress. And they are happy, for now, to settle for any relief their patients derive from psychopharmacological interventions.

In general, most of the practitioners I spoke with find antidepressants in particular helpful and even "lifesaving" for patients with severe illness like major depressive disorder, which often includes suicidality, one of the most dangerous symptoms to treat, for obvious reasons. Yet most of the Biodynamic and Psychodynamic practitioners also describe the 1980s as having ushered in an optimism about medications that was not entirely justified. While they all prescribe or refer patients for medications and report that they are useful in many cases, they are also often ineffective and occasionally harmful.

Furthermore, Dr. Kane (Psychodynamic) explains, it is not just a belief in biological etiology but also external forces at play that lead to an overreliance on medication. Of the centrality of medication, she told me:

> I think it is very problematic and I think it's driven by reasons other than actually what's helpful for patients such as insurance company reimbursement—this isn't something I've thought about a lot, it's not something I think about very much—the American Psychiatric Association, since that's their thing, medication is their thing, it may be a way of protecting the guild essentially, and insuring a livelihood for their members. . . . I think it's a problem for psychiatry in that psychiatrists coming up are not being trained to do very much psychotherapy and certainly not very much psychodynamic psychotherapy, so I think as I see it they're becoming almost robotic in a certain way.

Dr. Kane addressed a common sentiment among the Psychodynamic Psychologists, many of the Biodynamic Psychiatrists, and a few of the Biomedical Psychiatrists as well when she describes the external forces at play on doctors' decisions to prescribe medications. Moreover, she suggests that the pressure to prescribe medications also results in decreased odds of psychiatry residents being trained as what she sees as well-rounded clinicians. While she seemed to feel a bit uncomfortable levying this kind of critique, and she noted this "isn't something I've thought about a lot," she also seemed to have a fairly coherent notion that psychiatry training does not provide the tools she and other practitioners agreed are important to becoming an effective clinician.

Dr. Clarendon's (Biomedical), response to my question about etiology inadvertently offered insight into one of the other common concerns about medication—the uncertainty of the outcome. Dr. Clarendon treats a lot of teenagers, and sees 95 percent of her patients for medications alone. She described some of her skepticisms about medication:

> I think age and neurodevelopment is a tremendous factor. Quite honestly, I see people in their twenties who are anxious and depressed, and I know that for so many of these people they will just be different in thirty years. They will just be different. And that has to do with the fact that their brains are still myelinating. So, a lot of it is age, a lot of it is depending on the particular environment that the patient is in. Drugs and alcohol are a huge factor. And precipitating symptoms. I am often surprised that even now, I am not as good as I would like to be at that stuff. I don't think we really understand a lot of the causes of these kinds of illnesses. I am

not even sure that for the majority of patients that I see that to some extent that I am providing—yes the medications are helpful and yes the medications reduce anxiety, they improve mood in some cases they really dial down the intensity of terrible thoughts, suicidal thoughts—but I am not certain that in a different time, when there wasn't medications that these patients would come in to see the doctor and talk on a weekly basis and the thing would eventually run its course. . . . I really don't know. I mean, there is clearly a subset of people with moderate to severe depressive symptoms or perhaps some of the more severe kinds of obsessive-compulsive disorders where the medications are really making a substantial, substantial difference, and maybe left un-medicated those conditions would then become really life threatening. They would evolve and become very, very serious, but for a great many disorders, just not.

In Dr. Clarendon's language about myelination and neurodevelopment are clues to her biomedical thinking. Though she does not think symptoms are static, as is evident in her description of young adults who change over time and because of shifts in their environment, she supports the use of medications especially for severe symptoms. Many practitioners described similar murkiness in determining whether medications are indicated and effective, a sentiment expressed especially often by the practitioners who continue to see their patients in talk therapy while they take medications. As they come to know patients over time, it is sometimes unclear whether it is talk therapy or medication that has caused their symptoms to abate. Some practitioners pointed to the irony that while no one can predict how a patient will respond to medication, it is often seen as the go-to treatment.

I often encountered this sense of uncertainty not only about the mechanism by which medications work but also about whether they work at all. Responding to my question about what it's like to be in both the psychoanalytic and psychiatric worlds, Dr. Lewis (Biodynamic), explained that she has "more tools to look at things, and it's more fun also to step out" and "analyze a case from multiple perspectives." She offered an example:

I have a severe borderline patient who underwent ECT and all kinds of stuff. A complicated case and nothing helped, and no medications helped and I put her on another medication really without any expectation that this medication will do much else. And about a month after that medication was started she took a turn, but I will never be able to tell you what got her to take the turn. In fact, I think it's not the medication because she's going back to her old ways. I think it's been more the systematic interpretation and the work we've been doing, but you will never be able to purify it, and I think the way to see it will be if down the road a lot of her symptoms will be really gone for a really long time like a year or years as opposed to two months or six weeks. So, if I were a pharmacologist I would say she's responding to this medication. I would happily discharge her. I would happily just consult her once and then never see her again and have a conviction that this medication is wonderful for borderlines. Or if she were in a research study then she would be considered a responder and the study would be over there and they wouldn't know that the same woman two months from now will be struggling with the same stuff and eventually through the therapy she will actually climb out of it and I don't know. Maybe this is the miracle bullet.

Dr. Lewis chuckled as she uttered the words "miracle bullet." She was not shy in telling me she finds the idea that medicine can solve all problems ridiculous. At the same time, her commitment to helping her patient in whatever way possible means she would be happy if any of the treatment options worked, and she uses medications because she wouldn't want a patient to miss out on anything effective. There is broad consensus that combined treatments are the best bet partly because of the strengths of each model, but also because of the uncertainty of what will actually work for whom.

Talk Therapy

Psychodynamic Psychotherapy: "Being Open to the Uniqueness of a Person"

Unlike their descriptions of the use of medication, my interviewees who practice talk therapy did not have as concise an explanation of the role of talk therapy in their treatment. What was clear was that my psychoanalytically trained interviewees feel strongly that psychodynamic treatments are effective and offer patients a richer sense of themselves and their symptoms through the depth and intensity of the treatment, which they often describe as in large part related to the frequency of meetings. Talk therapy, particularly that which is psychodynamically informed, I was told, fills gaps that medication-based treatments cannot. This notion is perhaps clearest in Dr. Park's description of the different foci of the biomedical model and the psychoanalytic approach:

The DSM is precisely useful for grouping people, not for looking at aspects of concern that are necessarily N of 1. So, all sorts of things like meaning, character, personality, the soul, mind, and how it works are not involved in DSM. DSM is explicitly and purposely non-etiological so if you're at all concerned with etiology, DSM is not concerned with origins. Psychoanalysis and meaning, I would say has a drive toward the notion of origins, the origin of symptoms, the origin of—human experience in childhood, in trauma and various. We're interested. The DSM is not interested in that.

When Dr. Park says "we," she means psychoanalysts, which she uses to distinguish herself from Biomedical Psychiatrists—those whom Dr. Park links directly to the DSM. Psychoanalysis involves thinking about the various etiological factors responsible for her patients' conditions; an attempt to understand origins is much of her daily work.

Practitioners described treatment as helping patients gain insight and control of unconscious assumptions through an intense relationship with their analyst. Treatment is connected to ideas about etiology insofar as it offers clues to the patient's early life and particularly experiences with attachment figures. Yet the connection between treatment and etiology is complex for analysts, and the practitioners I spoke with were not always able to clearly articulate precisely how analysis works or what exactly causes the symptoms their patients experience. Dr. Gold (Biodynamic) explained that new patients often ask her "well what do you do?" when they first come in for treatment, to which she replies, "What do we do? What's my job? My job is to try to help you understand yourself." Even some of the Biomedical Psychiatrists who don't practice talk therapy described it as a way to learn about the self and rise to better functioning. As such, its goals are different from those of medication-based treatments. Dr. Haman (Psychodynamic) paused between thoughts and chose her words carefully as she described what she sees as the guiding principles of psychoanalysis:

Well, I think first of all, just the emphasis on depth. I was gonna say insight, but that almost feels like that doesn't quite capture what I'm trying to get at, but something about going into that kind of depth. And I'm thinking in contrast to the cognitive behavioral stuff where I'm gonna give you some exercises and I just want you to think about this and we're not interested in where this comes from or what this is about, we just want to fix it, change it. And I guess insight and self-reflection, and as kind of clichéd as it sounds, the—I still think there's something to helping somebody bring to the surface what's unconscious to help open up other possible ways of behaving and feeling in the world, which I don't think happens necessarily in other forms of treatment.

Dr. Haman again describes the focus on the unconscious, self-reflection, and insight as the key differences from other brands of treatment like psychopharmacology or more routinized talk-based treatments like CBT. Perhaps most concisely, Dr. Coffrey (Psychodynamic) told me that the uniqueness of psychoanalysis lies in its examination of unconscious conflict, through the relationship between the therapist and the patient. She described this as "the central focus of treatment." Specifically, she told me transference is what sets psychodynamic treatments apart from others, again marking the practitioner herself as an important tool in the treatment.[2] Dr. Brighton (Psychodynamic) echoes Drs. Haman and Coffrey when she describes the mechanism by which she believes psychodynamic treatments work: "It's the number of times you're seen per week. Frequency, frequency of treatment. The quiet of the analyst, the quiet of the analyst. The respect for the patient's conscious unfolding. What am I missing? It's really transference, countertransference, the frequency of treatment and the belief that what is curative is the interpretations that are made within the transference."[3]

In addition to the intensity and duration of the treatment, psychoanalysts often described the success of treatment as largely dependent on the analyst herself. Practitioners explained the crucial role of the practitioner in the psychodynamic approach as a part of its depth and intensity, as Dr. Adams (Psychodynamic) did when she told me what sets psychoanalysis apart from other treatments:

> It's meeting a person without preconceptions, being open to the uniqueness of a person, getting to know the person as an individual rather than a representative of a diagnostic category or any other kind of category, being open to getting to know yourself through the interaction with a patient, and work on self and with other being linked. . . . Which is what the unconscious is all about, right? The unconscious is the unexpected, so if you go into an interaction with a person in therapy or outside of therapy, feeling like you know what is going to happen or what should happen ahead of time, then that's inconsistent with any idea of the unconscious.

Dr. Adams is especially focused on the interweaving of the practitioner's and patient's consciousnesses as a tool of the treatment, which requires a proficiency and expertise derived from many years of training. Dr. Taylor explained that the function of the analyst is one of the most important characteristics of psychoanalytically informed treatments:

> The major principle of psychoanalysis is this principle of unconscious mental functioning, right? That the assumption that you have as an

analyst . . . is that your patient in front of you has expectations, wishes that guide their perceptions and their behavior that they may not be aware of. And sometimes in a helpful way, but often in a problematic way, and that is what your role as a psychoanalyst is—to help bring those to the fore, so that the patient can have a little more control.

Psychodynamic Psychologists in particular readily described the importance of the therapeutic relationship. To be adept at psychoanalysis requires arduous training and an ability to be deeply insightful on the part of both the practitioner and the patient. And sometimes, as Dr. Brown (Biodynamic) explained, the success of psychodynamic treatments is partly about "tenaciousness" and "not giving up and hanging in there with a patient for lengthy periods of time if necessary." It's a commitment on the part of both the doctor and the patient.

Because of its richness and depth, Dr. Nelson (Biodynamic) explains, psychoanalysis is a better choice for patients with certain kinds of troubles:

> So, in terms of psychoanalysis in my practice I see it as the way to offer the deepest treatment experience. And that it fits a niche in terms of treating people who are suffering from sort of coping problems and character problems. And that the group of people who would take advantage of it are often people who would also take advantage of other modalities so they may also use medications and other kinds of therapies before entering psychoanalysis, but that the psychoanalysis offers the most intensive, rigorous approach to personality and character problems and higher level neurotic problems for those who have the motivation to do it.

Psychoanalytic treatment has much to offer for people with what Dr. Nelson describes as "coping" and "character" problems, which are often attributed to environment rather than biology. Psychoanalysts often offered examples of specific patients for whom in-depth talking treatments have been hugely successful. While it is hard to re-create the most telling examples without violating the confidentiality of both my interviewees and their patients, here Dr. Gold (Biodynamic) describes her interaction with a young woman who came in for treatment of anxiety symptoms:

> [She] called herself a [specific kind of phobic]. She has a fear of [a behavior] and she went on the internet. People who have a fear of [that specific behavior] are getting themselves a diagnosis. She has an anxiety disorder and it's manifest in this way. Now what that phobia, what that anxiety is about will come over time. I've been seeing her for about two months and we've figured out one main reason, but most symptoms are

multidetermined . . . one of the multiple determinants for her is aggres-
sion. It's a way of expressing angry feelings. So, her fear [of engaging in
a certain behavior] near certain people in certain circumstances and not
in others—that's one that I assume as the treatment goes on we'll find
out other meanings for it too.

Dr. Gold's patient could have taken medication for anxiety symptoms, but her
goal is to help this patient understand the deeper cause of the symptoms and in
doing so hopefully assuage their severity or eliminate them entirely, offering her
what doctors describe as "control" or "freedom." Psychodynamic therapy,
Dr. Gold explained, involves the patient tolerating a process of looking into herself and being open to uncovering what is causing her suffering (and even the
suffering of those around her). Dr. Gold quipped. "You can't make an omelet
without breaking eggs." In order to feel better, the proverbial mental eggs have
to be cracked open and emptied, scrambled around, put back together anew—
albeit with many of the same fundamental ingredients. That, she explains, is
the goal of analysis.

When I asked Dr. Linden (Biodynamic) what she sees as some of the central contributions her field makes to society, she articulated two somewhat different accomplishments—one for the biomedical model and another for the
psychoanalytic:

I think much of my day is about people who are struggling and who are
suffering. I think there are many ways of addressing that. People turn
increasingly to a spiritual, religious variety, and people also turn to psychotherapy, so I think it's to relive suffering, both psychotherapy, as well
as the medication. And I would hope that in practicing medicine it's also
the purpose is to heal, so that's the big thing. . . . I think that a psychoanalytic frame provides a more deliberate approach to ongoing questioning, and that we don't know answers so easily. One can become seduced
if you have this antibiotic or that medicine, like we know. But the best
clinicians in medicine are the ones who know the field and are always
humbled. Like I'm always the most impressed by the internist or the surgeon who says, "Hmm, this doesn't add up," and knows the question to
ask. And so, to me, always learning something new is crucial, and that
when you are in private practice you are in a very privileged position to
being able to understand the individual, and that always pushes the enve-
lope from how that particular person is not fitting in to what you learned
in one way or another. It also should be an area of expanding knowledge
and research and contributing to society as a whole. It's a very big deal

for the public to know that schizophrenia is an illness. Bipolar disorder is an illness. This affects families. This affects people.

Dr. Linden is clear that the goal of both psychopharmacology and psychoanalysis is to help people with their suffering, and to help people "heal." In describing both the biomedical and psychoanalytic approaches as extending beyond clinical contributions, Dr. Linden articulates what many of her colleagues see as one of the defining features of psychoanalysis: it's richness, depth, and engagement of the patient in an exploration of the psyche. She also describes the "seduction" of the biomedical model as a somewhat false promise of a solution to symptoms that no one understands that well, but one that offers the illusion of scientificity, in part because of its link to diagnosis and biological etiology. She characterizes psychoanalysis, a field that provides "ongoing questioning," as something closer to an art form, and medicine more as a science, a common dichotomization.

One way practitioners described psychoanalysis was by explaining, as Dr. Ferris (Biodynamic) did, the different potential outcomes of medication treatment and psychoanalysis:

On the first layer of it, psychiatry has an enormous amount to offer to people who are psychiatrically ill with psychotic illness or with affective illness because we have such a huge armamentarium now of medications that simply was not there [when I was a resident]. Prozac came out just as I was finishing my residency. Prozac and all of those antidepressants have really revolutionized treatment and has made treatment much more available to so many more people. So, you know, I think from psychotic disorders to major affective disorders to chronic low-level depression and so on there's been huge change in treatment, and that change in treatment has made a lot of people more able to live their lives, better able to live their lives with much higher quality of life. But I also think paralleling that that analytic psychiatry and analytic psychology and psychotherapy—despite the fact that less people use it than they used to because of insurance reimbursement and so on—offers just as important things to people. I mean, when I think about what people have been able to do just in the years that they see me. I mean, I might not be able to treat as many people as an internist or as many people as a psychopharmacologist, but nevertheless make profound changes in people's lives when they're willing to look at the things that keep them from reaching their potential.

Dr. Ferris references the "psychiatrically ill" in noting the strengths of the bio-medical model and people who are "willing to look at the things that keep them from reaching their potential" as more appropriately under the purview of dynamic therapy. In describing why she feels her field is rewarding, Dr. Brighton (Biody-namic) also explained the advantages of psychodynamic treatment in terms of depth: "I think it's a gift to offer anybody the chance to get a grip on their uncon-scious destructive behavior, to think about the meaning and purpose of their lives, to dabble in freedom and choice. Those are just huge. Not to mention symptom relief, relief from day to day suffering. If you can be that person that helps with that, it's very nice." Dr. Brighton describes treatment as an experi-ence for both patient and clinician; the work can be rewarding for both parties. Psychoanalysts are deeply committed to using psychoanalytic principles in their practice and feel confident in its ability to help patients. In Dr. Brighton's statement that psychoanalysis "offers just as important things to people" as psychopharmacology, she alludes to the looming sense in the field that it is less valuable or less able to assuage symptoms. Biodynamic Psychiatrists were particularly attuned to this critique, and though they sometimes directly addressed this question about the worth and efficacy of psychoanalysis, they more often conveyed a subtle reaction to what they (and most psychoanalysts) see as a problematic cultural assumption that analysis is less valuable compared to the biomedical model.

But it is the very sense that psychoanalysis offers a richness to treatment and to understanding people more generally, coupled with its waning role in mainstream psychiatry that led many of the psychoanalysts, and even some of the Biomedical Psychiatrists to worry about the next generation of practitioners. Dr. Sullivan (Biodynamic), for example, referring specifically to child psychia-trists, described the deficit in psychodynamic training for today's residents: "The residents who I worked with this past year have really suffered and struggled with the absence of any of that kind of [dynamic] input. . . . People want to understand, even when they're medicating their patients, why they're compli-ant or not compliant and what's going on in the room."[4] Dr. Remsen (Biody-namic), who was a resident in the early 1960s, was already in practice during the paradigm shift and explained that she worried about "the devaluation of in-depth therapies, the overvaluation to some degree of medication, and the dis-paragement of in-depth therapy," which she told me is likely "one reason why it's undervalued." She explained, "There's some residency programs which don't even teach it, so how are you supposed to deal with patients? Patients all have dynamics; they all have histories." Particularly the practitioners trained in psychodynamic psychotherapy worry that without even some understanding of it, the ability for doctors to do their jobs well diminishes.

Though less frequently cited as a concern, Biomedical Psychiatrists like Dr. Clarendon expressed similar worries. She indirectly pointed to some of the forces that impacted her own cohort, students who began their residencies just before 1980, as she explained her concerns about residents:

> I don't know that residents are really taught or given the opportunity or experiences to try and understand their patients in terms of the, this is a hackneyed word: holistically. I think too often, because of the way that residents are taught to think about psychiatric illness, because of the time pressures, because of the way that residents are taught to document, I think there's an insufficient appreciation for the fact that people are not their illness and that you can be afflicted with depressive symptoms, or bipolar disorder, or schizophrenia, or panic disorder, and that is one aspect of that person's experience, that patient's experience. But you really have to understand much more about that, and to be able to really put those symptoms in a context such you can be maximally helpful to the patient.

While they certainly do not have the same allegiance to psychodynamic ideas or practice as their analyst colleagues, Biomedical Psychiatrists understand that exposure to some psychodynamic training is helpful even for a largely psychopharmacological practice. And in their discussion of what current residents and trainees lack is clear insight into the reasons they value psychodynamic psychotherapy, a topic I return to in the conclusion.

"Good Bedside Manner Stuff" versus Deep Exploration of the Psyche

Despite shared concerns about current residents' lack of skills in anything beyond diagnosis and psychopharmacology, and the recognition that training in talk therapy is helpful, there is a crucial difference between Biomedical Psychiatrists and their psychoanalyst counterparts in their descriptions of talk therapy. In detailing the importance of exposure to both models in training, Dr. Brooks (Biomedical) explained, "Given that most patients would arguably benefit from both, I think to have people trained in both is important. And some of the psychotherapeutic stuff is related to good bedside manner stuff, so it's probably techniques and methods and partly an awareness of a set of human issues." Dr. Brooks summarized the way the majority of the Biomedical Psychiatrists described the influence of psychoanalysis on the field—it helps psychiatrists to be better at talking with patients. But they rarely describe it as a treatment paradigm that stands on its own. When they refer to talk therapy, psychodynamic psychotherapists or psychoanalysts mean something much richer than "an awareness of human issues." Consider this interchange I had with Dr. Hart (Biomedical) when I asked if she sees any patients strictly for medications:

Dr. H: I never see people in and out five minutes for meds. I never do that. Even people who I see three or four times a year for medications are typically people who maybe we had something more intensive going, they're stabilized, or they're in a joint treatment with someone else for meds. But when I do see people for medication, my shortest visit I offer is a thirty-minute because I feel like, the medicine, I have to take into account the context of the rest of what's happening in their life. I'm not strictly biological in the sense that I think a pill is going to be a fix-it for people.

DS: So, in that thirty-minute visit, is it talking about symptoms, or . . .

Dr. H: It's symptoms, it's about medical, you know, have they had any changes in their medical status. But, you know some will come in and they'll tell me they're very anxious. Okay, so what is that anxiety all about? Well, it turns out the anxiety is that they're not getting along with their spouse, and so we talk about what is happening there, how are they dealing with things, do they maybe need to do some couples work, is it about their own personality characteristics that are contributing? Because I like to educate the patients that I don't truly think that you take a pill and it fixes things, I don't.

Dr. Hart is clear that she's not interested in just "five minutes for meds." She doesn't consider herself a psychopharmacologist and considers all her sessions talk therapy. Yet 90 percent of her patients take medications; only 10 percent of her practice is made up of patients who are not on any medication, and her patients in talk therapy alone come once or twice a month, or in rare, special cases once a week. This is very different from what analysts mean when they say "talk therapy"; even though Dr. Hart cares about the circumstances in which patients' symptoms present, her conceptualization of talk therapy is to ask about relationship issues or other aspects of current life context, and possibly to work with patients on personality issues, but her sessions are not long enough and her meetings not frequent enough to make deep connections between the past and present. Despite any psychodynamic training, Biomedical Psychiatrists generally practice a basic form of talk therapy, but it is qualitatively distinct from that of their psychoanalytic counterparts. Some Biomedical Psychiatrists may be informed by dynamic principles and may see patients more regularly than the average biomedical practitioner, but the depth of the treatment is nowhere near as great as that of their psychoanalyst colleagues who have years of training in psychoanalytic theory and practice.

Some Biomedical Psychiatrists were attuned to the differences between the kind of talk therapy they provided and a deeper analytic treatment. Dr. Sutter told me that she practices both psychopharmacology and talk therapy, so I asked if she considers both types of treatment with all patients, to which she responded, "I did my residency in places with very dynamic, and I know enough about dynamic stuff that I feel very comfortable sort of dealing with the dynamics to a certain degree, but if someone's really interested in sort of more psychoanalytic psychodynamic treatment, I'll refer them." Dr. Sutter wanted me to know that she's familiar with in-depth talk therapy and that she doesn't ignore issues of deeper meaning in her practice. She explained that her residency mentors in the 1980s impressed upon her the importance of psychodynamic treatment. She sees most of her patients once a week, which is unusual for the average Biomedical Psychiatrist. Dr. Sutter has about seventy-five patients in her practice, and she told me she sees 25 percent just for medications. Everyone else she sees once a week, and many of the medication-only patients are former therapy patients, so she knows them reasonably well. Though she says the main kind of therapy she practices is cognitive behavioral, her practice is smaller and she talks much more about what she describes as "long-term relationships" with patients than many of her Biomedical colleagues. Though she thinks more dynamically than the average psychiatrist and she is not strictly a psychopharmacologist, even Dr. Sutter's talk therapy is dramatically different from the descriptions of psychoanalysis we heard earlier from both Biodynamic and Psychodynamic practitioners. On one hand, psychodynamic principles and certainly classic psychoanalytic practice are largely on the periphery of the field. On the other hand, the recognition that the therapist (even in psychopharmacology) is a figure of meaning to a patient does represent retention of some very basic guiding principles of psychoanalysis.

Limitations of Psychoanalysis

Many of my interviewees praise in-depth talking treatments and lament their loss in mainstream psychiatry. Yet the lack of evidence for its efficacy in an evidence-based profession leaves practitioners, especially those trained in psychodynamic treatment, frustrated both at the second-class nature of talk therapy compared to psychopharmacological treatments and at the uncertain efficacy of their treatments (which they are often careful to remind me is also true of psychopharmacological treatments). Dr. Haman (Psychodynamic) described "this tension" and "this problem" for psychoanalysts in "being able to demonstrate it as an effective treatment in some scientific way." She continues, noting, "a lot of debate in the field . . . is this a science? Or is this something like a science? Is it an art, and if it's an art, then how do you justify it as a treatment? And like all of that stuff I think is problematic. It loses some of its legitimacy in a way, not among those of us who are converts, but out in the press you definitely get that sense in the world that if there was more of a way to demonstrate its effectiveness in some scientific way, that it would help the field." Dr. Haman captures a common philosophical question about what, precisely, psychoanalysis is, but her fear is that this does a disservice to the field by making it feel like talk therapy doesn't live up to a standard of scientificity that may not be an appropriate bar against which to judge it. Yet there are substantive critiques often related to its limited application. Dr. Park (Biodynamic) described her circuitous route to psychiatry as one that she always knew would lead to psychoanalysis, as she is deeply connected to psychoanalytic theory and treatment. Despite her almost magnetic pull to the field, she also offers the most forceful critique of psychoanalytic practice:

> It is as a clinical endeavor in practice limited to very few people. So, who am I? I'm a person who tunes up Rolls-Royces basically. That's my job. . . . How many people can you see in your lifetime if you're seeing them three, four, or five times a week for a number of years? So, if that's an important part of psychoanalysis, the frequency and duration and depth, clinical psychoanalysis has to be in any immediate doctorly social sense relatively unimportant. So, it's a slow process, it's an uncertain process, unlike medication. Medication you come in with a panic disorder and you've got an 80 percent chance of responding and psychoanalysis I tell people it's gonna be burdensome in terms of time and money and it's gonna be uncertain in terms of results. Freud advertised psychoanalysis at the end of the last chapter of *Studies in Hysteria* for psychoanalysis as the goal of it was to achieve . . . what is the phrase? Everyday unhappiness. So how many medical specialties, how many religions inscribe on their banners "Come here and we will provide everyday unhappiness"? But that's psychoanalysis—that's what psychoanalysis has on offer. It should be a hard sell, all right. And these days it is. I have no quarrel with that, actually.

In describing what psychoanalysis does, Dr. Park is also clear about its shortcomings, particularly when compared to the biomedical model. I suspect a number of the analysts I spoke with would take issue with Dr. Park's notion that their work is equivalent to performing maintenance on expensive cars or that the analytic side of their practice doesn't have the ability to lead to important and lasting change, even if it is for wealthy, often well-resourced populations, but overall, she corroborates some of the usual critiques of the field, which are often aimed at classic analytic practice. Dr. Park highlights a common, competing feeling for analysts: on one hand they would ideally like to see an integration of psychodynamic ideas with mainstream psychiatry, while on the other they recognize that everything from the appropriate patient pool to the notions of etiology are different, often at odds, and likely impossible to integrate.

Many of the critiques of psychoanalysis are related to what Dr. Adams (Psychodynamic) describes as being "out of sync with the culture. . . . I think psychology markets itself now," she explains. "Psychology has a marketing orientation. It's trying to get into the health care system and market itself as efficient in a particular way, and so cognitive behavioral kinds of therapies fit very well with that kind of mentality. Psychoanalysis probably has ignored marketing kinds of consideration to its own detriment . . . there's been an arrogance in the field, like we don't have to publicize or justify ourselves or whatever, we just sit in our offices and do our thing." While there is an effort to change psychoanalysis's public appearance by adapting it to fit into a short-term model comparable to CBT, which a handful of practitioners mentioned, there was also a sense that psychoanalysts as practitioners, and even as researchers, have not managed to create a coherent presentation to the public that fits with the broader cultural norms, both within and outside the mental health fields. When I asked Dr. Adams why she thinks cognitive behavioral therapy is so popular right now, she told me, "I think it fits very well with a culture that probably is breaking down at this very moment, as we speak, which is very pragmatic and bottom-line-oriented, like, what's the measurable outcomes? Kind of an antiromantic attitude in the culture at large, like, you fly in an airplane and you see all these guys on their laptops with spreadsheets and all of that. Cognitive behavioral therapy fits much better when there are measurable goals, outcomes, short-term, cost efficient, that kind of mentality." Psychodynamic Psychologists generally pointed to mismatches between the culture and an in-depth, talk-based treatment model rather than actual problems with the paradigm itself. Some critiqued classic psychoanalysis for letting people suffer unnecessarily, as Dr. King did in the opening of this book.

In general, analysts' critiques of their field concentrated on problems specifically related to how limited the application of psychoanalysis is, how unpredictable its duration will be, and how uncertain the outcome can be. Dr. Sullivan (Biodynamic) explains, "Psychoanalysis is a very particular treatment that requires both commitment, time availability, enough of a sense of a frustration and current difficulties that it requires a whole confluence of things to make it the treatment of choice. I think probably more people would benefit from it than actually can, you know just in terms of logistics, manage it." Dr. Sullivan highlights what many of her psychoanalytic colleagues describe as one of the limiting features of the practice for both practitioners and patients: time and money. At the time of our interview, most analysts only had a handful of patients in psychoanalysis largely because of financial constraints. Dr. Sullivan had seven analytic patients, the most of any of the practitioners I spoke with. Though seven analytic patients may not sound like a great number, it means twenty-eight "hours" of work per week. When patients are in analysis, they usually pay a reduced fee. If, for example, a practitioner charges three hundred fifty dollars per session for a regular visit, she might charge two hundred for an analytic session since there are four sessions per week. Even the reduced fee is a great deal of money for patients, yet potentially not enough for a practitioner to support a practice in New York. At the same time, Dr. Sullivan prescribes medications—about a third of her practice is made up of medication-only patients. She sees the remainder of her patients for psychodynamic psychotherapy, often twice a week. Psychodynamic Psychologists often have very few patients in traditional psychoanalysis because of the time and cost—they cannot supplement their income with medication patients—though they see the majority of their patients multiple times per week and use psychodynamic principles in all their treatments.

Finally, practitioners described the waning demand for psychoanalysis as a problem for its continued role in the field. Dr. Gold (Biodynamic), who trained in the 1950s, during the height of psychodynamic influence, alluded to cultural notions that more immediate alleviation of symptoms is preferable over treatment that might require months or even years in order to see some progress— an accurate assessment of psychoanalysis in most cases. She says she witnessed "cultural shifts" in which "people are less willing to come four or five times a week and apply themselves diligently to understanding themselves." She continues, "People seem to want quick fixes. I think the drug companies have added to people's wish fulfillment that a magic pill will solve all their problems." Most of my interviewees noted a number of cultural factors that influence both practitioners and patient demand for psychoanalysis, psychodynamically informed treatment, and even infrequent talk therapy. Though it was at a reduced fee, psychoanalysts were required to pay for their own analysis. Practitioners have a sense that it is taxing for patients to pay even for infrequent treatment, and while most agree that patients are less willing to come in for talk therapy and that this has something to do with a "quick-fix" mentality, they also recognize that "will" is much more complicated than it may appear. Practitioners' and patients' concerns, which are intricately tied to managed care, lead to a preference for seemingly efficient, evidence-based treatments over those that seem uncertain and are time-intensive.

Dr. Remsen (Biodynamic) thinks that, beyond time and money, there is "less of an interest in the general population in in-depth, long-term exploration of psychic issues," a widely shared sentiment among the psychoanalysts. She doesn't blame this entirely on biomedicine, but regardless of the cause, she feels a poignant disinterest in and "devaluation" of the psychodynamic approach:

> I think a lot of psychiatrists and psychoanalysts have found that there's some patients who can benefit from twice a week psychotherapy perhaps as much as they can from four or five time a week psychoanalysis. That is kind of a critical thing to say [of psychoanalysis], but I do think that it's true. The other thing is finances and insurance coverage. I think one reason that a lot of people in Europe, for example, are in psychoanalysis—in Germany, I think, and some of the other countries in Europe have much higher percentages of people in psychoanalysis— is because it's covered by insurance. . . . Whereas here, I think you have a cap and if it's psychoanalysis, you get nothing, and people are not willing [and she later recognizes that most patients may not be able] to pay the price, and psychiatrists have to earn livings, especially young people starting out with a lot of medical school debt, families—they want to live a little bit.

Dr. Remsen attributed the dwindling use of psychoanalysis to a number of troublesome forces from both within and beyond psychiatry. In her description of the impact of financial factors and insurance coverage is also a straightforward critique of the frequency of sessions in classic forms of analysis. There is an underlying but telling theme in my conversations particularly with Biodynamic Psychiatrists about the troubles with the classic four-times-per-week iteration of psychoanalysis. While a number of practitioners described the value of twice-per-week sessions or indicated that they consider three-times-per-week sessions to be analytic treatments, it was hard to tell if analysts truly feel that these modified treatments are as effective or if they are a response to constraints like insurance and patient demand. Reality is likely a combination of the two. It is notable that the mention of treatments with fewer sessions was always in the same breath as discussion of the changing culture around treatment or managed care.

As a result of a culture that favors short-term, medication-based treatments and strict limits on coverage for talk-based treatments, patients often do not even really know what psychoanalysis is—even those who seek out talk therapy. Though the majority of my interviewees deny that patient demand has had an influence on the likelihood that they will prescribe medications, they recognize that patients do not often come into their offices with a clear idea about what psychoanalysis is. Consider this interchange I had with Dr. Mill (Biodynamic) when I asked what usually leads people into treatment:

Dr. Mill: Even in New York, it's been my experience that very few people come in requesting psychoanalysis. I have had that experience a few times, but they're such special situations. . . . People connected with the training institute might be interested in analysis or friends and partners of candidates studying analysis may want an analysis. They want it for themselves or their partner wants them to. So, I've had people come in and say I want analysis but it's very rare.

DS: What is it about analysis, do you think, that attracts them?

Dr. Mill: It's interesting because they don't necessarily—you know, they have an idea of what analysis is or even sort of a fantasy that may or may not actually resemble what analysis is. I would say not, usually . . . but they do have a sense and a desire to understand themselves in a deeper way and they do have an idea that analysis, more than the other treatments available, is supposed to provide something, somehow, in some way, of exploring themselves or knowing themselves in a deeper way. . . . I think I would say it's a little more self-knowledge than symptom relief. Although sometimes their symptom is the pain and or the suffering they have from the sense they have that they don't know themselves or they can't understand why they're in this situation they're in, more than depression or anxiety or drug use. . . .

DS: And, so on the other hand [for psychiatric treatment], it would be the symptoms?

Dr. Mill: Most people come in because they're unhappy and that's kind of different. The people who come in specifically for analysis, although that's a tiny number, don't necessarily say "well I'm just really unhappy." They're often really confused. They really don't understand themselves.

It is difficult to sustain an analytic practice when people don't ask for or even know what psychoanalysis is. This is true even of practitioners: Biomedical Psychiatrists generally don't know enough about it or find it relevant enough to critique. Psychodynamic Psychologists shared some of the concerns about time and cost but were relatively uncritical of psychoanalysis, which is likely attributable to their singular training in that model (which often began in graduate school, before psychoanalytic training). The Biodynamic Psychiatrists, who treat a significant number of patients using their psychopharmacological training (with the exception of those who trained before the 1980s), were the clearest about the shortcomings of the analytic model; their training in both models often allowed them to feel at home critiquing both. And while all the psychoanalysts I interviewed felt the field offers significant relief to patients and a depth of self-exploration not available elsewhere, they also recognize some of the reasons why it remains an uphill battle for it to have a significant impact on mental health practice more broadly, particularly given the dominance of evidence-based thinking and the sense that the biomedical model offers more reliable symptom alleviation.

Different Treatments, Different Goals

All of my interviewees either prescribe medications or refer patients for them, yet there are some essential differences between the Biomedical Psychiatrists and my interviewees who are psychoanalytically trained. In my early interviews with the Biomedical group, I was used to talking to Biodynamic Practitioners who spoke often about the role of both medication and talk therapy in treatment and pointed to the necessity of both. I approached my initial interviews with the Biomedical Psychiatrists with many of the same questions, such as what role they think medication plays in treatment, a question that was often met with lengthy responses from the Biodynamic Psychiatrists, but when I asked this of the Biomedical Psychiatrists they frequently looked confused and responded with something along the lines of "it *is* treatment" or in one case even "I'm not sure what you mean." I continued to ask the question even though it often created an awkward moment, and despite realizing after the first few interviews that it was really an almost absurd question to ask someone whose practice revolves almost entirely around prescribing medications.

Recall that Dr. Evans, whose practice is largely psychopharmacological, told me she couldn't identify any negative aspects of the shift toward the biomedical model in psychiatry. Of her training in the 1980s, she told me she "got in at the right time" because the field was newly focused on biology and medical interventions, specifically noting a better understanding of the brain and medications. On the other hand, even Biomedical Psychiatrists can be much more amenable to psychodynamic psychotherapy if their training offered them some significant training in the approach (either formal course work or mentorship). Dr. Morris, for example, who finished medical school and moved into her residency years in the early 1980s, described her psychiatry training as psychodynamic and identifies herself with the "old-fashioned people." Though she "is grateful there are psychopharmacologists out there," she uses medications more sparingly, which is evident when she says, "I think it's irresponsible to treat patients with medication alone initially."

Ultimately, all my interviewees agreed that there is a qualitative and quantitative difference between symptoms that are minor troubles and those that are severe enough to require medication. They all allude to the twin pillars of DSM diagnosis: severity and duration (criteria not only for diagnosis but for prescribing medications). Most of my interviewees also referenced some version of the appropriateness of a symptom or the context in which it occurs, though Biomedical Psychiatrists were most likely to focus on symptoms, the presence of which is sometimes enough (regardless of why they emerge) to warrant the prescription of a medication. After all, most patients who wind up in a Biomedical Psychiatrist's office are there precisely because they or another mental health practitioner believes their symptoms warrant medical intervention. This is not necessarily the case with the Biodynamic Psychiatrists, even though they have a license to prescribe medication, or for the Psychodynamic Psychologists, who would have to refer to achieve a combined treatment. Medicine is often only one part of a treatment for analysts, who feel deeply connected to the practice of talk therapy even if they also feel strongly that medications are an important tool of their trade. Despite this, Biodynamic Psychiatrists do see patients for medications only—in fact medication-only patients make up a significant percentage of their visits, on average 56 percent of their patients, which is about the same as for their Biomedical Psychiatrist counterparts. However, the comparison is unfair given that Biomedical Psychiatrists are much more likely to define even an infrequent patient as a combined treatment, whereas the Biodynamic tend to think of infrequent patients, even those they see every month mostly for mediation check-ins, as medication-only patients. As such, a fairer comparison might be the number of patients *not* on any medication, which is an average of 39 percent for the Biodynamic and 12 percent for the Biomedical.

Like their feelings about the DSM, practitioners' attitudes toward medication are complicated. Aware of the critiques from outside the field and the perils of a treatment lauded as more efficacious than the research and their own anecdotal evidence sometimes bear out, my interviewees had plenty of criticism, especially for overprescribing. Many are wary of treatment exclusively with psychopharmacology. And at the same time as practitioners across all three groups agree that severity (and often duration) is a reasonable indicator for the use of medication, whether psychopharmacology should be used as a primary form of intervention is intricately linked to practitioners' varying notions about the causes of the symptoms their patients bring to treatment. The extent to which practitioners believe in biological etiology impacts their feelings about how useful medications are and how many of their patients are prescribed psychotropic medication. For the Biomedical Psychiatrists, the average percentage of patients who take medications (including patients who are in combined treatments) is 88 percent compared to 62 percent for Biodynamic Psychiatrists and 43 percent for Psychodynamic Psychologists.

With the exception of those who trained before the 1980s, the psychiatrists I spoke with tended to privilege biology in their etiological considerations, which makes sense given their training. In her ethnography of psychiatric training programs, anthropologist T. M. Luhrmann (2001, 30) informs us that "what residents actually learn is to do what they have to do: admit, diagnose, and medicate patients, and—less pressing these days, see them in psychotherapy." Practitioners are trained in thought communities (Fleck [1935] 1979) that provide different schemas for understanding patients and their troubles (Smith and Hemler 2014). In other words, as Luhrmann (2001, 83) explains, "in both of these approaches, the biomedical and the psychodynamic, what one learns to do affects the way one sees." Practitioners trained in psychodynamics will see complicated relationships and unconscious motivations, whereas those trained in the biomedical model will see clusters of symptoms and family patterns of illness. As they move into their practice years, psychiatrists trained after 1980 (and some before) remain committed to the use of medications in part because they've seen them as helpful and believe that their patients' symptoms operate at the level of neurochemicals. Psychodynamic Psychologists also think of etiology as multidimensional, but tend to privilege psychological and interpersonal factors over biology; when practitioners think of troubles as born of the mind and environment, they are less likely to see medication as a necessity or as a central part of treatment at all. However, it is of note that treatment is also driven by the division of labor in the mental health fields today, which means that regardless of practitioners' thoughts about etiology or appropriate treatment, patients have been less likely since the 1990s to look to psychiatrists for talk therapy (Shorter 1997).

Though psychopharmacology and psychoanalysis were highly separate practices until just a few decades ago, today combined treatments are widely thought to be an effective form of treatment (compared to either talk therapy or pharmacotherapy alone), particularly for depression (Pampallona et al. 2004; Cuijpers et al. 2009). For the Biodynamic Psychiatrists especially, the notion that etiology is biopsychosocial allows practitioners to feel it is appropriate to use a combination of medicinal and talk therapy treatments, both of which they are trained to practice, and which sets them apart from the Psychodynamic Psychologists and the Biomedical Psychiatrists. Though medication and talk therapy are used together frequently, the way psychoanalysts talk about the drive to understand origins also indicates somewhat different goals of the two brands of treatment, and different kinds of patients may make use of each type of treatment. The goal of psychopharmacology is to reduce symptoms, while psychoanalysis is much more focused on deep understanding of the self, particularly of unconscious forces. While insight is believed to lead to symptom reduction, diminishing symptoms is not the only explicit goal. What is also clear in my interviewees' narratives about medication is that the rationale for the use of combination treatments is at least somewhat rooted in uncertainty about what really works. With practitioners not knowing in many cases whether it's the medication or the talk therapy (or a combination of the two) that is effective, it makes logical sense to use them both to get the most benefit of treatment possible.

In the end, numerous forces support the use of medication, and even analysts, practitioners who were once the most resistant to the use of psychopharmacology, think of medication as a catalyst for talk therapy. Very few of the practitioners with whom I spoke, across all training backgrounds, support the use of in-depth talk therapy as a sole mode of treatment when patients present with serious symptomatology. Perhaps most illustrative of this is that significant percentages of Psychodynamic Psychologists' patients take medications. Within mainstream psychiatry, the basic principles of psychoanalysis are still considered important by some, but the depth of the treatment and the focus on the unconscious are largely absent from the Biodynamic Psychiatrists' practices. Even psychoanalysts have limited numbers of patients in classic psychoanalysis; often, they opt for psychodynamically informed psychotherapy in two-times-per-week sessions, and sometimes settling for once-per-week treatments, as

Schechter (2014) notes when she wonders why practitioners train in psycho-analysis at all today given the inability to maintain psychoanalytic practices. The varying belief and training in the biomedical model and likewise varying belief and training in psychoanalysis have ramifications for practitioners' experiences of their work and deep consequences for their identity as professionals, topics I turn to in chapter 5.

The Consequences of the Biomedical Model for Practice and Practitioners

Psychodynamic Therapy in a Biomedical World

Dr. Brooks was the first Biomedical Psychiatrist I interviewed. Her practice is small mostly because she focused increasingly on research after her residency, which makes her an anomaly among her Biomedical colleagues. Yet she enjoys treating patients and described a long-standing interest in the mind that extends to her college years, when she decided psychiatry was an apt fit for a student interested in both biomedicine and the humanities. As we discussed her training, Dr. Brooks described the typical factions between psychoanalysts and what she calls "biologists" that characterized the 1980s watershed decade in psychiatry and her training years. I asked her whether she thinks those tensions persist, to which she replied,

> I think that psychoanalysis still has influence. It's a question of relative degree. If you look at, generationally, older psychiatrists, there were still some, decreasingly so, who were trained primarily as psychoanalysts. And you know, I would argue that psychoanalysis still has important roles, and I would say most psychotherapy is still psychoanalytically rooted to some degree. There's been spinoffs, and we know that for a lot of conditions the best treatment is a combination of therapy and something biological. . . . I think there are probably still a few ideological biologists who argue biology is the answer period, but I think that most people in practice would probably sense that you need both, and part of that is the wide range of psychiatric disorders, some of which are gonna benefit more from one or the other. . . . So, it's not like we found the

schizophrenia gene or the depression gene and it seems, at least to my
sense, that we probably won't. In other words, we might be thinking you
have a predisposition, but the genetics is suggesting there's a mix of environment, genetic loading, and then environmental factors. So, the notion
that just one approach is the answer I think is gonna be harder to maintain probably because I think the science is bearing that out.

Dr. Brooks doesn't think the tensions she witnessed in her training persist
because she senses less intensity on both sides; there are fewer ideological biological voices, and despite the dominance of the biomedical model, she feels
like psychoanalysis still has some basic influence on the field. Dr. Brooks alluded
to conflicts between psychodynamic and biomedical psychiatry largely as historical or part of her own autobiographical account of training. Though she later
explained that "ideological biologists" remain and can be problematic, her overall assessment was that the clashes of the 1980s have faded, a common view
among the Biomedical Psychiatrists I interviewed. And though she never trained
in in-depth talk therapy of any kind, insofar as the science bears out its utility,
Dr. Brooks considered psychodynamic treatment to be a worthwhile part of a
combined treatment. Despite operating within a much more biomedical framework than their colleagues of past generations, I rarely heard Biomedical
Psychiatrists express hostility toward any form of talk therapy including psychoanalysis or its practitioners. In general, they mentioned the importance of
the basic principles of psychodynamic treatments mostly in terms of their com-
plementarity to psychopharmacological treatments.[1] Biomedical Psychiatrists' practice is in line with the dominant treatment approach in the field, and
when I asked them about tensions in the field or paradigmatic clashes, they
rarely conveyed concern and often had little to say.

The story is more complicated for practitioners whose treatments are exclusively or even largely psychodynamic or psychoanalytic; when they described
what it's like to be a psychoanalyst in a biomedical world, they used terms like
"exhausting," "difficult," and "hard to integrate." This chapter focuses on the experience of practicing psychoanalysis in a biomedical world, which offers insight
into the tensions many practitioners face given the structural and cultural conditions under which they find themselves practicing. While I have resisted
grouping practitioners by their training beyond the portraits in chapter 2, here
it is appropriate to do so, as the experiences of practicing under the influence
of the biomedical model vary widely between the Biomedical Psychiatrists and
the psychoanalysts, and even between analysts with different training and professional credentials.

Biomedical Psychiatrists

Dr. Clarendon, the only insurance provider I interviewed, echoed Dr. Brooks's description of the staunch divide between practitioners in hospitals in the 1980s:

> When I went to medical school, and when I was in residency, there was at that time kind of a war between the psychoanalytic camp and the eclectic camp, and when I interviewed for residency programs this was what people talked about—was this a psychoanalytical or was this a biological program? If you went to residency at Wash U, you were going to a biological program, if you did your residency, at the time at Sinai, which is no longer the case of course, it was a psychoanalytic program. So that's gone, no one talks like that anymore.

As many practitioners did, Dr. Clarendon offered a retrospective account of the paradigmatic clashes and divisions between particular institutions, and within the field more broadly, which she characterized as having been between the "psychoanalytic camp" and the "eclectic camp." Though she clearly identified the split as having been between "psychoanalytical" and "biological" training programs, she seemed to have a sense that psychiatry in the 1980s was characterized by a divide between psychoanalysts and everyone else. When Dr. Clarendon explained "no one talks like that anymore," she was referring to the descriptions of programs as either Biological or Psychodynamic. It is tempting to hear her claim that people rarely refer to training programs in this language of past divisions in the filed as a kind of détente, a proclamation that the clashes or even the basic tensions between psychoanalysts and biomedical practitioners are a thing of the past. Especially in the context of Dr. Brooks's claim that the staunchest biological critics have softened or even disappeared, it often sounded like she and others were indicating that these paradigmatic silos of the past no longer exist. Yet when I asked the majority of the Biomedical Psychiatrists how they would characterize psychiatry, they used the words "Biological," "Biomedical," and even "symptom-based prescribing." And when they described the field in general, they were clear that most training programs today are also biomedical. When they talked about the common brands of talk therapy, they referenced CBT and dialectical behavior therapy (DBT), and only a handful who had some psychodynamic training in their residency mentioned psychodynamic psychotherapy or psychoanalysis. In other words, the fading tensions are more an indication of the biomedical model's victory over psychiatric training and practice rather than a diminishment of tensions between the models.

Though it seemed ironic at the time, I was also regularly told that "most psychotherapy is still psychoanalytically rooted to some degree," as Dr. Brooks explained. By this, she and her colleagues typically meant that the basic notion that the relationship between practitioner and patient is central to the treatment and that the context of people's lives is important. A legacy of the Freudian era, these ideas impact most practitioners, even those whose talk therapy sessions are infrequent and generally revolve around medication management. For the Biomedical Psychiatrists I spoke with, psychoanalysts are not the enemy. They are not seen as an opposing camp. And psychodynamic principles are not a challenge to the practice of Biomedical Psychiatry. Biomedical Psychiatrists like Dr. Doughty even expressed concern at the "move away from the richness of getting to know your patients" because she told me she thinks "included in psychodynamic principles is sort of in-depth training on how to interview a patient." Even the Biomedical Psychiatrists sometimes lamented the loss of what they think are the basic lessons of psychoanalysis, yet their practice is largely in line with the medical model; beyond a template for talking to their patients and situating their lives in a larger context, psychodynamic principles don't play much of a role in their practice. Biomedical Psychiatrists practice medically in a medical world. A multiple-session-per-week therapy that focuses on deep meaning and the relationship between the patient and practitioner was largely irrelevant for Biomedical Psychiatrists; depth and transference, which psychoanalysts overwhelmingly described as the key guiding principles of psychodynamic treatment, did not figure in a typical session for Biomedical Psychiatrists and weren't concepts they typically encountered in training or thought applicable to their own practice.

Although some, like Dr. Clarendon, whose practice is largely psychopharmacological, see a handful of patients for what she calls "longer, more in-depth psychotherapy," she is up against structural constraints that prevent longer or more frequent sessions. Dr. Clarendon reserves two or three hours a week for psychotherapy patients, and although she says she would like to practice more psychotherapy, she explained that she needs to see three patients per hour both because of pressure from insurance companies and to make enough money to live and work in one of the most expensive cities in the United States. Dr. Clarendon also explained that she has read extensively about how to bring in some conversation beyond symptomatology even for her shortest medication management sessions since she points out that "you really have to understand much more about that and to be able to really put those symptoms in a context such that you can be maximally helpful to the patient." In other words, she believes it matters to understand patients beyond their symptoms, but even as one of the

Biomedical Psychiatrists who seemed most committed to the importance of context and getting to know her patients, she does not see many psychotherapy patients, both because of external constraints on her practice and because of her training.

The majority of the Biomedical Psychiatrists I spoke with simply did not raise any issues when I asked them about psychoanalysis or other forms of talk therapy, though some Biomedical Psychiatrists occasionally alluded to continued tensions between the Biomedical and Psychodynamic paradigms; a handful described psychoanalysis as "elitist," too slow, or unable to treat certain kinds of severe illness (the very problems many of the analysts I interviewed also identified). Dr. Hart, who supports the use of psychotherapy only for less severe conditions, told me "what really scares" her is that there are "a lot of people out there, not so much psychiatrists, but I think social workers and so forth who are treating some very sick people and sometimes . . . therapy alone is not appropriate for that." She sees psychiatrists as better equipped than nonmedical professionals to treat "very sick people." And she assumes that it is only the nonmedical practitioners who would be less discerning and treat someone who she indicates would need medication with talk therapy instead. Not only are the paradigmatic divides clear here, but there is a notion that psychiatrists are better trained and more discerning.

Perhaps the clearest example of the way Biomedical Psychiatrists seemed to think about the field was when they indicated the need for psychiatry to move even more toward neuroscience and evidence-based medicine. The only Biomedical Psychiatrist to point directly to current tensions or conflicts in the field was Dr. Elm, but rather than pointing to clashes between biomedical psychiatry and psychoanalysis or other forms of talk therapy, her thoughts turned to what she described as a significant issue between psychiatry and neuroscience. When I asked her what she sees as the dominant paradigm in psychiatry today, she responded as follows:

> I would say basically twentieth-century philosophy or nineteenth-century philosophy is the dominant paradigm. I think that phenomenology outweighs science in psychiatry. That science research in psychiatry is really crappy, primarily oriented towards the pharmaceutical industry, you know, and doesn't really take into consideration the larger concepts of what's going on. I think that psychiatry is way behind neuroscience by and large—not entirely, but certainly in practice and that either there's the world of psychoanalysts, some of whom are interested in neuroscience and trying to integrate it, but still in a paradigm which is early

twentieth century. And I think then there are the psychopharmacologists who are in a science paradigm that's not very well integrated with what's going on in the world of science.

For Dr. Elm, the key issue is the lack of integration of psychiatry with what she sees as "science." According to her, analysts are stuck in the early twentieth century and psychopharmacology isn't real science—at least not yet. By comparing the mental health fields to other branches of neurochemical and science, Dr. Elm points out that psychiatry aligned itself with neuroscience using psychopharmacology, but with few reliable tools or evidence of neurochemical or biological etiology. The tension in the field today, in other words, is about whether psychiatry is evidence based enough; Biomedical Psychiatrists may recognize the value of psychodynamic treatments, but when they think about key issues in the field, they look to the future and the potential for psychiatry in evidence-based medicine and neuroscience, rather than to past debates, which Dr. Elm sees as miring the field in philosophy. Of course, many of the same practitioners also point out that even neuroscience involves a certain amount of "early twentieth-century" thinking.

Biomedical Psychiatrists of the 1980s actively sought dominance for their brand of treatment in hospitals that were run by psychoanalysts, many of whom were openly hostile to the use of medications. Yet the Biomedical Psychiatrists I spoke with do not see psychoanalysis as a threat today and psychoanalysts do not appear to be perceived as competition. In addition, they appear to value certain psychodynamic principles; for example, they see the context of their patients' lives as important, and they tell me they work to establish a rapport with patients. They were clear that both are important in order to be a successful practitioner, but they rarely ever mention key psychodynamic principles like the impact of unconscious factors or the complexity of the patient's perception of the context. Psychoanalysis as a treatment paradigm is largely irrelevant to their practice, and even when, for example, patients are in a psychodynamic treatment with another practitioner, that talk therapy is typically seen as an addendum to psychopharmacology. The psychodynamic model is not really a true contender in terms of what they see as tools used in mainstream psychiatric treatment. And there is little indication that they make much of a distinction between psychodynamic psychotherapy and any other kind of talk therapy.

Although Biomedical Psychiatrists currently practice within the dominant paradigm, they do experience various conflicts. Throughout the book I have pointed to some of their fears about overmedicalization, pigeonholing, loss of context, and overly diagnostic and psychopharmacological psychiatry training. Yet they are biomedical practitioners in a biomedical world, and for most whether or how to integrate psychodynamic principles into their treatment is not of concern. Even if they think a patient is an ideal candidate for talk therapy, they can easily refer the individual to another practitioner and retain the psychopharmacological part of the treatment for themselves. In fact, Dr. Hart explained that she feels "really fortunate" to know and work with colleagues who "consider themselves at home using multiple treatment models," and whom she describes as doing "terrific work" of combining "therapy" and "meds." She explains that she thinks these colleagues are "psychodynamically informed, but they're also pretty cutting edge with medicine as well." Though she clearly thinks that having an advanced understanding of psychopharmacology is a prerequisite for good practice, she's open to what she calls "therapy," which she uses as shorthand here for "psychodynamically informed" treatments.

In short, the Biomedical Psychiatrists I spoke with seem to regard the tensions between the psychodynamic and biomedical paradigms and their practitioners as largely a phenomenon of the past. Yet the narrative, particularly around what it's like to work with practitioners from different training backgrounds, was dramatically different when I asked psychoanalysts about their experiences. Particularly analysts who trained before the 1980s described the remaining issues with the biomedical model taking over, and still often experience it as encroaching on psychodynamic thinking. For all the analysts I spoke with, working with practitioners who are not trained analysts or who haven't had any exposure to psychodynamic principles can even be confrontational. And because psychoanalysts practice in a much less evidence-based model, where they are often forced to defend their practice and theoretical beliefs, they are more attuned to the remaining paradigmatic debates and tensions that were carried into the twenty-first century.

Biodynamic Psychiatrists

Biodynamic Psychiatrists regularly practice psychodynamic psychotherapy—not just talk therapy, but intensive, often multiple-session-per-week treatments. Due to time and financial constraints, most limit their more traditional four-times-per-week psychoanalytic patients but see a significant number of their patients twice a week (some even three times), a standard frequency for talk therapy among practitioners trained in psychodynamic psychotherapy. And their psychodynamic training shapes the way they think about patients, even when they are strictly psychopharmacological. While practicing both psychopharmacology and in-depth talk therapy is relatively uncomplicated for most,

Biodynamic Psychiatrists generally recognized the tensions between the two paradigms in terms of their etiological considerations and treatment goals; for some practitioners, this translated to cognitive or psychological conflict, and most experienced at least interpersonal tensions when interacting with other practitioners, mostly those with strictly biomedical training. In short, they experience a range of consequences to practicing psychoanalysis and psychodynamic therapy in a biomedical world.

The Challenge of Expertise

One of the key trials of having a foot in both psychoanalysis and psychopharmacology—what some Biodynamic Psychiatrists describe as having one part of the brain that's focused on meaning and one that's focused on diagnosis—is the feeling that they can't be equally good at both brands of treatment. After 1980 psychiatrists who trained in psychoanalysis felt the push and pull of competing expectations, and many felt pressure to be able to perform both treatments well. Dr. Nelson explained that while she doesn't think it's impossible to be good at both, "it depends somewhat on how hard you can work and how easily these things come to you." She continued, "For me, really learning how to get good at psychoanalysis has taken a huge amount of work and it would be hard for me to also put the work into keeping up on the cutting edge of pharmacology at the same time. And I think there are people who maybe the analytic things come more easily and maybe they work more and go to both, keep up with both sets of meetings, but I really have found it hard to do both." Dr. Nelson appeared wary as she explained what I heard from a number of Biodynamic Psychiatrists, particularly those relatively junior in their field; because their psychiatry training was largely biomedical, they have had to work against their rigid training in categorical thinking and medical diagnosis to become good psychoanalysts. But as they do, they are also working against the dominant treatment modality in their field and sometimes against their identity as psychiatrists.

Older Biodynamic Psychiatrists, having trained before the biomedical shift, do not describe the need to be all things to all patients; they manage the issue of expertise by limiting their use of medications or by not prescribing them at all. Dr. Carroll, one of the most senior, for example, explained that she chose talk therapy over psychopharmacology: "So when the new medications came, and then one medication after another, I felt that I couldn't spend all my time reading all these medication publications, so I found a good psychopharmacologist and I referred my patients who needed some pharmacological help to the psychopharmacologist while I continued to work with them [in talk therapy]."

Dr. Carroll accepted that she would refer patients for medication, especially when it was a difficult case, because it felt impossible to be as good at both kinds of treatment. Furthermore, Dr. Carroll became a psychiatrist at a time when psychodynamic thinking dominated residency programs, so she feels much more at home treating patients in psychoanalysis than with the use of medications, and she had little to no training in psychopharmacology. Regardless of age or cohort, however, most of the Biodynamic Psychiatrists recognized the difficulty of being good psychopharmacologists and psychoanalysts. Yet the majority prescribe medications, unless they encounter a really difficult case, when they sometimes refer patients to a more specialized psychopharmacologist. Despite the challenges to their sense expertise because of their dual training, their practice remains largely unaffected.

The Freedom and Frustration of Dual Training

The issue of expertise is intricately tied to professional identity.[2] A handful of the Biodynamic Psychiatrists like Dr. Lewis said they feel like they can move fluidly between their role as psychopharmacologist and psychoanalyst. She told me, "I think I just have more tools to look at things and it's more fun also to step out and try to look at [patients' problems]." But most Biodynamic Psychiatrists described a closer alignment with one paradigm or the other. Their professional identity is largely shaped by the period when they trained as psychiatrists and psychoanalysts. Given their lack of training in the biomedical model, most older Biodynamic Psychiatrists have largely psychodynamic practices. Those over sixty were in their residency years during an era when their psychoanalytic training was essentially a deeper exploration of concepts they learned in their residency years rather than two different models. Of the Biodynamic Psychiatrists, seven trained squarely in the psychodynamic era: three were in their late sixties, one was in her seventies, and one was in her eighties. Three were approximately sixty at the time of our interview, which means their residencies would have been in the 1970s, but their early practice years would have been right on the cusp of the biomedical shift.

The oldest Biodynamic Psychiatrists sound a lot like Psychodynamic Psychologists in most regards. When I asked Dr. Gold why she decided to train in psychoanalysis, she told me,

> At the time that I trained—I'm seventy-one—really psychoanalysis was at the pinnacle of psychiatry. Biological psychiatry was really just beginning. The antipsychotics were just beginning to come to use, that plus sleeping pills and I guess Milltown was just in its heyday, right? And so

my own experiences got me interested in psychoanalysis and the orientation of my teachers was psychoanalytic and I wasn't interested in treating chronic psychotic patients. It didn't seem like it was very interesting
or challenging personally. It didn't suit me. Psychoanalytic exploration
of the mind did.

Dr. Gold's medical school and residency years were squarely in the psychoanalytic heyday because of her cohort. At the time she trained, there was a very
limited use of psychopharmacology in large part because the biomedical model
was not yet developed. As such, she considers herself a psychoanalyst and
applies that model in all encounters with patients. She identifies deeply as an
analytic thinker. However, even she sees a handful of patients for mediations
only, which she writes off as essentially "wish fulfillment" for her patients—it
satisfies an unconscious desire but doesn't do much in terms of actual treatment—
and she was clear that for the profession more generally, she sees psychopharmacology as a financial boon, and not much more. She described colleagues
whose practices are largely psychopharmacological: "For most people, I mean
it's a great way of making money, but it isn't very interesting. If you're interested in making money, that's what you do, and there are a lot of people doing
that, but it's not very challenging. That's my opinion, personally." Dr. Gold had
two patients in traditional psychoanalysis at the time of our interview, and she
dedicates a lot of time to teaching and supervising analysts in training, which
is a key part of the job for many senior practitioners. The majority of her practice
is two-times-per-week psychodynamic psychotherapy.

Similarly, Dr. Carroll, whose residency was in the 1950s and analytic training in the early 1960s, had little exposure to psychopharmacology in her training years because, in her words, "there was no psychopharmacology, hardly
any, just some heavy tranquilizers and they were experimenting with antidepressants." Like Dr. Gold, Dr. Carroll "farms out" her patients to psychopharmacologists when they need medicines because she believes that depression, a
condition she often treats, is a "biological illness." While most analysts believe
depression is complicated and not attributable to one factor alone, it was not
uncommon for Biodynamic Psychiatrists to describe it in biomedical language.
Dr. Carroll is somewhat less skeptical of psychopharmacology and biological
etiology than Dr. Gold, yet because of her cohort, she too is not trained to prescribe medications and therefore feels more comfortable letting other people,
mostly more junior colleagues, do that work. She told me, "Well, basically, I
identify myself as a psychoanalyst, and I let the pharmacological community—I
farm out my patients to that—I don't want to deal with the side effects and what-

not, let them talk to Dr. X." The older analysts can be quite critical of the centrality of psychopharmacology to the field, and they describe this as frustrating, yet even when they recognize deep divides between the models, they remain identified as analysts. Their medical training puts them in a position to make a choice about how much (if at all) they want the biomedical model to figure in their practice, and generally it's very little.

An exception to the rule, Dr. Dean, who was in her late sixties at the time of our interview, offers insight into the power of training and mentorship. She told me despite the era in which she trained (1970s), she "had very good training in psychopharm, even though it was just an infant science at that time." This is likely why she feels strongly connected to other physicians, which was evident when she told me, "If people ask me what I am, I say I'm a physician first, I'm a psychiatrist second, and a psychoanalyst third." She was also clear that prescribing medications was always "a very important part of the work," which she connected to her thinking about etiology. She explained, "I always felt that—and Freud believed that too—eventually we would change the brain, we just didn't know how to do it, but we would do it chemically. He always believed that." Her description of her alignment with the biomedical model felt almost ironic, as she uses Freud's sometimes very basic biological ideas to support her own allegiance to medications. Dr. Dean sees patients for medications only, which accounts for a little less than half the patients in her practice, and which is more typical of younger analysts. While it may seem as though Dr. Dean is at odds with Drs. Carroll and Gold, who more closely align with the psychoanalytic part of their training and practice, what the three share in common is that they all align more closely with one model or the other. Unlike their Biomedical counterparts for whom psychoanalysis is mostly outside the jurisdiction of their practice, the Biodynamic group operates within two very different treatment approaches. Most explain that their dual training gives them the freedom to use both models, but most also feel more closely aligned with one paradigm over the other, which is in line with their sentiments that it's challenging to be equally good at both.

More than half of the Biodynamic Psychiatrists I spoke with trained in or after the 1980s. The very chance of a psychiatrist deciding to train in psychoanalysis today—to spend an additional five years training in a model that's not in line with what's dominant in the field—is slim. All the Biodynamic Psychiatrists had some exposure and allegiance to the psychodynamic model before or during their psychiatry training; some had mentors in their residency who communicated its importance or had parents or other important figures in their lives who were analysts and exposed them to its utility. For example, Dr. Sullivan told me of exposure to Freudian ideas in high school and of classmates whose parents were analysts. And Dr. Halsey's parents are analysts, which sparked her interest in dynamic ideas. Despite her allegiance to the biomedical model, she told me that her residency was not "very good," which to her meant it was too biological, so it was her parents' friends and colleagues who helped her to see another side of the field. Dr. Dean told me she read Freud in a college course, and when she did her residency there were supervisors who, she explained, "felt like they had gone to my office and read my notes the night before . . . the good ones were the analysts."

The younger cohorts of Biodynamic Psychiatrists are much more aligned with the biomedical model. While they too spend five years in analytic training after their psychiatry training, which they value greatly, their primary professional socialization is in a biomedical framework, and their psychoanalytic training, while it may radically alter their thinking, does not necessarily change their practice all that much. In other words, though they describe an allegiance to psychoanalysis, the current cohort of practicing psychoanalysts was trained first to use the biomedical model. Dr. Warren, whose psychiatry residency was in the 1990s, explained,

> The people who taught me psychoanalysis are not as pure psychoanalysts as maybe is traditionally thought. They're psychiatrists for the most part, and their feeling is, for example [senior Biodynamic Psychiatrist] . . . she diagnoses first. She uses DSM. She uses medications with kids. She's not so different from me in that regard. Yes, there are some times where someone's coming in who's just analytically out there for me. . . . I feel like one of the things that gets really frustrating for me is analytic treatment for kids with autistic spectrum disorders. Not to say that a very high-functioning Asperger's kid [can't benefit from analysis]. But you know, come on.

Dr. Warren doesn't feel much tension between the two models because she sees herself as a hybrid practitioner who practices within the biomedical model, but who also draws from her psychoanalytic training, which is how she describes the mainstream model for Biodynamic Psychiatrists today. When she points out that she and one of her mentors, a well-respected practitioner in her circle, treat kids with medications, and her "frustration" at the idea of treating a child with autism with only psychoanalysis, she's pointing to classic critiques of psychoanalysis, but arguing she doesn't need to levy those critiques because no one practices that way anymore. In short, she was telling me not only how she fits in with other analysts, but also that the notion of using psychoanalysis as a sole treatment model, as something "pure," even for the generation of Biodynamic Psychiatrists before her (practitioners who trained in the era just prior to the 1980s), is not common practice. Dr. Warren regularly sees patients, the majority of whom are children, for medications only. She also practices in-depth talk therapy with about 50 percent of her patients, but does not currently have any patients in a traditional psychoanalysis, which is in line with how she was taught—by psychiatrists who use psychoanalytic principles, but who also practice a great deal of psychopharmacology.

In fact, Dr. Warren explained to me that she trained in psychoanalysis mostly to be "a better dynamic therapist" because she didn't feel equipped for such an endeavor after psychiatry training. It seemed to me that her intention was not necessarily to practice psychoanalysis per se, and as such, her training in its principles shapes her thinking, but need not present her with any real conflict; she doesn't see herself as having to choose one model or the other, and her treatment is never purely psychodynamic. In describing their identity as practitioners, whether they align more with the psychoanalytic or biomedical model or whether, though less common, Biodynamic Psychiatrists tended to see themselves as a true hybrid, their descriptions of these allegiances almost always elicited a discussion of the contradictions between the models, and sometimes with the practitioners who practice differently than they do.

Difficulty in Integrating the Models

One reason why practitioners often align themselves with one paradigm more fully than the other is that it's hard to have a foot in both worlds, as Dr. Warren explained:

> The analytic training for me was about being a better dynamic therapist. I think it is a hugely helpful thing in my work on a day-to-day basis, but the complicated part is often in talking to colleagues who haven't had the training and, when I'm at [Institute] doing analytic stuff I can sort of speak in one way and if I'm talking to child psychiatrists I'm gonna not go into too much detail about the dynamics. . . . If you split it off too much then the people who don't have the analytic training don't learn anything in that regard and the people who think too analytically don't get challenged about the medical part, so you try to kinda bring both in but it's sometimes, it can be exhausting for one thing.

In these descriptions it's also clear that Dr. Warren feels her psychoanalyst and Biomedical colleagues are in somewhat different worlds, rarely exposed to competing ideas. Biodynamic Psychiatrists sometimes feel like they have an obligation both to push psychiatrists to think psychoanalytically and psycho-analysts to recognize the biomedical, which means a sort of constant vigilance and awareness of the tensions between the models. While having both models available was widely described as beneficial for practice because it offered an enhanced toolkit, it can also cause internal conflict, as Dr. Nelson explained:

> I think [psychoanalysis is] very difficult to integrate with the medical model. And since I see the medical model as my bible, it's always chal-lenging for me to be an analyst because I'm constantly going in the other direction when I do analysis. So, the hard thing for me is that medicine, being a doctor, is very much focused around alleviating suffering and helping people rise to function and analysis is much more about digging up and uncovering and opening up material that's deep and that it doesn't always immediately in the short run make people feel better. So, I see a lot of contradictions in integrating it.

Many of the contradictions Biodynamic Psychiatrists experience are internal, a result of extensive training in one model that offers deep analysis, and one that focuses on eliminating symptoms. Dr. Nelson explains that the models have sig-nificantly different treatment goals that are not entirely compatible.

Interpersonal Tensions

Some of the Biodynamic Psychiatrists experienced more concrete, interpersonal tensions, like Dr. Halsey does, when she encounters mainstream psychiatrists, whose thinking is rigidly diagnostic. She explained she finds them "just very hard to deal with," and told me it's like an encounter with an internist, where she has to be "very straight to the point, very concrete: these are the symptoms." Dr. Halsey and others described a need to interact with practi-tioners in different ways depending on whether they are trained in psycho-analysis or not.

Some analysts feel that there is an almost confrontational, unpleasant exchange between mainstream psychiatrists and analysts. For this reason, Dr. Mill describes that being a member of both the psychoanalytic and psychi-atric communities can be trying. In reference to a previous comment she'd made about moving between the analytic and psychiatric communities, Dr. Mill told me, "I certainly wish it was something we could all fluidly navi-gate, and I fear it is not. In child psychiatry there's no relationship at all. In fact, if you're an analyst you're sort of dismissed and rejected." A number of Biodynamic Psychiatrists felt that they were sometimes pushed to stay within the biomedical paradigm so as not to risk critique or even ostracism. Dr. Taylor explains that she hasn't personally experienced the more extreme forms of bias against psychoanalysts, but in the field at large, she thinks it "can be problematic":

> I live in a city where there's relatively greater acceptance of psychoanal-
> ysis. In the program that I trained in, psychoanalysts were very respected
> so I've not found it to be particularly problematic among psychiatrists.
> But I do believe that people elsewhere have problems with that feeling
> that their views—perfectly valid views—are kind of dismissed based on
> a bias against psychoanalysis. They maybe would be less likely to get
> referred a patient, a patient who might benefit from that approach because
> of a bias against it, but I actually don't experience it that much.

Though she has not felt bias directed at her because of her analytic views, many of her colleagues, also analysts in New York City, have. It is of note that when Biodynamic Psychiatrists talked about tensions in the field for psychoanalysts, they rarely considered their Psychodynamic Psychologist counterparts, focus-ing instead on other Biodynamic practitioners although, as I discuss shortly, it is the Psychodynamic Psychologists who feel most poignantly that they are taken less seriously and that their experiences more generally are ignored.

Though it is mostly the more senior analysts—those who did not train extensively in psychopharmacology and the diagnostic model when they were in residency—who regularly refer their patients to other doctors for medication management, most Biodynamic Psychiatrists consult specialists particularly when they encounter a difficult psychopharmacological case which again con-firms the difficulty at being expert at both models. Biodynamic Psychiatrists have a strategy for referrals that allows them to avoid as much conflict as possible. Dr. Elliot explains, "The people I try to use are people who are either them-selves psychoanalysts or have some education and openness to the psychologi-cal in a person." They worry Biomedical Psychiatrists might focus solely on symptoms and disease and consequently not see the patient holistically. Dr. Lin-den, perhaps most directly, explains the difficulties in professional relation-ships when she describes being part of both the psychoanalytic and mainstream psychiatric worlds: "I think amongst some people it can feel very polarizing . . . and I think there's still certainly that group within psychiatry that feels that many injustices and things were done poorly by psychoanalysts,[3] but also people . . . have, I think, legitimate complaints for those who only see people as moving molecules, which is obviously not the case." She reiterates the sense that analysts are held accountable (by Biomedical Psychiatrists) for all the ste-reotypes about their field and practitioners in it, for instance, that they are

elitist and rigid and that they are against treatment with medication and biological thinking. Dr. Linden also pointed out that the biomedical group risks
"pigeonholing" their patients, rather than seeing them as unique cases; at the
same time as they are aware of tensions with Biomedical Psychiatrists, they also
critique what they see as an overly medicalized field and practitioners who they
sometimes describe as lacking nuance. Because they have a foot in both worlds,
they risk tense encounters on both sides.

While the majority of the Biodynamic Psychiatrists experienced some kind
of tension at either the cognitive or the interpersonal level, some did not. For
instance, when I asked Dr. Dean if she has any trouble navigating between the
psychoanalytic and the mainstream psychiatric communities, she told me, "I
don't because I have colleagues who are like myself." Part of not feeling much
tension between the two models for her is spending time with colleagues who
are like her, and because she can and was trained to prescribe medications, she
rarely has to navigate relationships with people outside her professional worldview if she chooses not to. This is especially important for Dr. Dean, who
trained in the 1960s and 1970s when Biomedical Psychiatry was "an infant science." Because she has a more psychopharmacological practice than most of
her generation of psychoanalyst colleagues, which, again, she attributes to "a
very good training in psychopharm," she has a lot of autonomy and control over
all the moving parts of a psychiatric and psychoanalytic practice. When Biodynamic Psychiatrists were able to limit their interactions with strictly psychopharmacological practitioners, they rarely encountered trouble, and they were
able to do this for the most part.

Given their training in both psychopharmacology and psychoanalysis, the
Biodynamic Psychiatrists I spoke with generally expressed strong attachment
to both models regardless of whether they privileged one over the other in practice. Like their Biomedical counterparts, the extent to which their residencies
were dominated by the biomedical model varies based on the era in which they
trained (pre- or post-1980s) and the mentors who most impacted their thinking;
most of the Biodynamic Psychiatrists experienced primary professional socialization under the guise of the biomedical model, and so they identify as medical
doctors. At the same time, they dedicated a minimum of five years to studying
and immersing themselves in psychodynamic theory and practice and were in
analysis themselves, usually for five years. So, it was not unusual for Biodynamic
practitioners to tell me that they do not, for example, attend the annual meetings
of the American Psychiatric Association because they don't feel aligned with
mainstream psychiatry, but regularly attend the American Psychoanalytic Association's meeting. Or they do not read much mainstream psychiatric literature,

but they do keep up with what's happening in psychoanalysis. Compared to their Biomedical counterparts, the Biodynamic Psychiatrists are much more attuned to what they see as a richness and broad benefits of psychoanalysis, not just in terms of how they relate to their patients and understand the context of their lives, but as an effective treatment modality that they think offers many patients the best chance to assuage or even alleviate symptoms, usually in combination with the use of medication. What makes the Biodynamic Psychiatrists unique is their larger toolkit; that it contains psychopharmacology allows them to treat a wide range of patients in a manner in line with biomedicine. With the exception of some of the oldest analysts, most feel at home using both the psychodynamic and biomedical models. While most also recognize they are trained in two very different treatment approaches, their dual training also allows them not to have to engage with nonanalyst practitioners if they don't want to, something Psychodynamic Practitioners are not able to avoid as easily, or sometimes at all.

Psychodynamic Psychologists

Psychodynamic Psychologists are not medical doctors; psychopharmacology is not part of their treatment toolkit, and their primary socialization is not in the biomedical model. Their work is largely psychodynamic psychotherapy and psychoanalysis, which many describe practicing under the thumb of the biomedical model. Compared to their psychiatrist counterparts, they experience the most conflict of any of the practitioners I spoke with, as a consequence of living in a biomedical world as nonmedical practitioners. In particular, encounters with psychiatrists around referrals are points of tension, although other professional encounters at conferences or in classrooms can also be difficult.

Dr. Brighton, who described herself as a "classical psychoanalyst," captured the "broad general tensions that exist between the groups" when she pointed to the hierarchical nature of encounters with psychiatrists:

> Psychologists will complain that MDs will see themselves as the gods who know it all and diminish or look down upon or talk down to the psychologists. And the psychologists, not understanding the medications when they have to deal with psychiatrists, often play into that view. That's how the psychologists view the psychiatrists as, you know, superior, playing God, diminishing them. . . . Many psychologists feel that they get dismissed as not knowing anything, they get overridden, that their treatments can get taken over by the psychiatrists, they'll send someone for a consultation. . . . I don't work with anybody who does this—I

have my own people who I feel close to who work collaboratively—but the complaints tend to be that the psychiatrists can dominate and take over the treatment.

Recall that Psychodynamic Psychologists are careful to refer to people with a "sense of psychodynamics," a central strategy for existing in a medical world as a nonmedical practitioner, the same strategy used by older Biodynamic Psychiatrists, who, because of their lack of psychopharmacological training, prefer not to prescribe medications. Even more junior Biodynamic Psychiatrists (who are highly trained in psychopharmacology) sometimes need to send a patient to a specialist for complicated cases, and also prefer to refer to someone sympathetic to psychodynamic thinking. Yet the central difference is that though the Biodynamic Psychiatrists may occasionally experience tensions in encounters with Biomedical Psychiatrists, they never worry their treatments will be taken over by another practitioner or that they will be seen as a less-than-qualified practitioner, an oft-cited fear that Psychodynamic Psychologists, who are considered lower in the hierarchy than Psychiatrists in the mental health professions, regularly have to manage. Dr. Brighton, who trained in psychoanalysis in the late 1990s, described these tensions as being outside her own experience—for other Psychodynamic Psychologists—which is clear in her use of the third person. She also indicated that she has her "own people" for referrals and highlighted the importance of avoiding practitioners who might treat her as inferior because she's a psychologist or who might think radically differently about the patient. She also suggested that psychologists "play into" the notion that they are uninformed or inferior because they don't understand medications. I did not get the sense that Dr. Brighton meant to blame her colleagues for their lack of exposure to psychopharmacology, but she did seem frustrated.

Indeed, some of the Biodynamic Psychiatrists confirmed the Psychodynamic Psychologists' fears. Though none explicitly denigrated psychologist analysts, Dr. Plymouth (Biodynamic) captured the sense of being better equipped in a broad sense. She described the benefits of being an analyst:

> It makes me a minority in the psychiatric community, which is something that I kind of like. I'm not sort of being a mainstream psychiatrist, and it means I have something to offer in psychiatry that not so many other people have to offer. In psychoanalysis—I became a psychiatrist because I thought there were advantages to being a psychiatrist and then becoming a psychoanalyst. I still think it conveys certain advantages and I like that I'm a psychiatrist rather than trained differently, as much as I value other sorts of training in psychoanalysis as well. It brings a certain bio-

logical perspective to psychoanalysis and I feel like I understand the medical orientation in psychoanalysis and that's important within the community of American psychoanalysis. . . . There are two different sets of advantages. There's this kind of biological and clinical kind of value . . . because I think that understanding people from a nonpsychological perspective is very useful in psychoanalysis. But then also administratively, organizationally, politically within psychoanalysis, the American Psychoanalytic Association as a whole, I think being a psychiatrist confers certain advantages in terms of understanding how people approach things.

Even as one of the handful of Biodynamic Psychiatrists who became a doctor with the idea of being an analyst in mind, Dr. Plymouth sees an observable advantage to being a psychiatrist in a biomedical world and not having to refer her patients to another practitioner for (the most socially sanctioned) part of a treatment, but also in bringing a medical perspective to bear on analysis. Dr. Plymouth's intention was not to suggest that Psychodynamic Psychologists or other nonmedical analysts are inferior or less valuable to the field, but in her description, there is also a clear sense that being a psychiatrist is more useful—perhaps even preferable—to being a psychologist analyst.

The Trouble with Referrals

The feeling that they are considered somehow lesser than was sometimes visceral in Psychodynamic Psychologists' descriptions of their encounters with psychiatrist colleagues. Most would rather refer their patients for medication consultations to fellow psychoanalysts or, at the very least, someone who understands psychodynamic thinking; not only do they feel this is best for the patient, but it also reduces the chance of having to deal with psychiatrists who are strictly biomedical and might introduce conflict into their treatment, especially by overmedicating the patient. Even Dr. Coffrey, who worked in a department of psychiatry for many years and therefore has an understanding of medications, chooses her referrals carefully:

> If I had my absolute choice, it's a psychoanalytically informed or psychoanalytic psychiatrist. And not because they know necessarily more . . .
> I might actually know a lot in the sense of what could help the person or various things. . . . And then I worry when it goes to psychiatrist X that that person has got to have a sophisticated understanding [of the patient], or otherwise, we're going to be at logger's head because they're gonna overmedicate, which is usually what happens, and/or skew things with that patient.

Dr. Haman was likewise keenly aware of the troubles with referrals. She explained that one of the big problems is it was sometimes not possible to refer to a psychoanalyst, leaving Psychodynamic Psychologists to settle for a Biomedical Psychiatrist—hopefully one with basic psychodynamic training. Dr. Haman explained that "the people who are psychoanalysts are not so keen on doing psychopharm [alone],[4] so even though in some ways there's something appealing to me about referring to them, they don't see themselves, their forte, as being psychopharm, so that probably isn't the greatest referral, but it does help to have them have some kind of sense of psychodynamics." Recall that many of the Biodynamic Psychiatrists describe having to give up some of their psychopharmacological specialization to become expert at psychoanalysis. Therefore, they may not be the best referrals when a Psychodynamic Psychologist is looking for someone who specializes in medications. The pool is quite small for a referral that is, on the one hand, not so specialized in psychoanalysis that they are less adept at psychopharmacology and, on the other hand, not so medically minded that they would be entirely unschooled in or even adversarial to psychodynamic principles. This means there is ongoing potential for tension in encounters with psychiatrists. It is also possible that patients come into psychodynamic treatment already in treatment with a psychiatrist, in which case a psychologist may have no control over these encounters.

In their descriptions of referrals, fundamental differences in ideas about etiology and the efficacy of medications are also clear. Dr. Livingston explains the need to be sure that the doctor to whom she sends her patients for medicines has an awareness of the person in terms of something beyond a body incubating an illness, one of my interviewees' common critiques of the biomedical approach. Dr. Livingston works with a lot of people who are diagnosed with personality disorders, which most practitioners agree are the most difficult to treat. For this reason, she says,

> it's good to have psychopharmacologists who are, who know how to work with those people because it can be really dicey and there's a lot of placebo responding and there's a tendency to overmedicate because they only have partial response to medications, so you just keep adding and adding and before you know it, the person's on like five medications and none of them are doing anything. Ultimately, you're, you want to work with people who know about—a lot of them are like my old supervisors and people who I know, have trained [in psychoanalysis] so we have a similar mind-set around medications.

Patients who have personality disorders (which psychoanalysts commonly treat), I was told, might respond in unpredictable ways to medications (regardless of what the actual effects of the drugs are), so it is very important to Dr. Livingston that the psychopharmacologist has an awareness of the patient's personality, psychological functioning, and atypical reactions to medications and the possibility that a single diagnosis does not fully capture the overall picture.

Sometimes Psychodynamic Psychologists were forthright about needing to feel a sense of camaraderie and professional similarity to the psychiatrists they send their patients to. For example, Dr. Kent described referrals:

> I have my people . . . I mean I'm still looking for the perfect one. But I look for people who are not like the many that I've encountered, who have no interest in having a discussion about the patient, and don't really understand the idea of the therapy, and often kind of impinge on the therapy. So, people who are more psychodynamically oriented, but it depends because if it's a very complicated case in medical terms, my first priority is that it's somebody who's very skilled with that disorder, like Bipolar Disorder or something, and I'll work around that.

Dr. Kent sends the average patient who needs a referral to her Biodynamic colleagues. But if a patient needs a specialized psychopharmacological consultation, a Psychodynamic Psychologist may not be able to get around the tensions or outright clashes with a more biomedically oriented practitioner in doing what's best for the patient. Referrals require careful planning, and attempts to minimize possible conflicts with practitioners who think and practice differently than they do.

The Psychodynamic Psychologists have only some control over which psychiatrist prescribes medications for their patient. Referrals create an ongoing potential for tension. Consider the following interchange I had with Dr. Butler about medication referrals:

> Dr. B: I send most of my patients to a colleague who's a close friend of mine who is a psychiatrist and an analyst, and so is sophisticated about therapy and analysis and so on. And we know each other very well so she knows— you know, some psychiatrists are very interfering and condescending. I think you have to find one you really get along with or a few that you really get along with who will do their job without trying to interfere with treatment.

DS: Condescending in the sense that . . . ?

Dr. B: That they think they know best. And I generally don't run across that because I have a choice of who I refer to, and I know them well, but occasionally it happens. . . . I remember there was one occasion where the psychiatrist was so intolerably controlling and interfering that I said I would never accept a case medicated by that person again because it was just impossible. I mean, essentially, she was doing a sort of parallel psychotherapy, and it was extremely annoying, and I talked to her about it, and she completely didn't see that. She was totally unapologetic and she knew best. Luckily the patient moved to another state and the situation was over.

Though Dr. Butler chuckled at the absurdity that it took something so drastic, like a patient moving away, to resolve the conflict between her and this Biomedical Psychiatrist, she was visibly annoyed as she recounted this experience. Her professional authority and her relationship with the patient were all challenged by having to deal with this outside interference in her treatment. Though she described this as "occasional," I heard these concerns repeatedly from Psychodynamic Psychologists.

"What You're Doing Is Bullshit . . . It Doesn't Make Any Sense"

It is not just in the context of referrals or encounters with psychiatrists around specific patients that tensions arise. In presenting her work to nonanalyst audiences, Dr. Sutton explained that she used to experience heavy critique; now she avoids those meetings altogether. As a seasoned analyst, she has more control over where she presents her work. She explained, "Twenty years ago, yes, I had to do that, and I did it. But you know, for example, I know that if I go to certain meetings, if I present my work, I will be attacked. I don't do it. I don't have to do it. This is my freedom. This is my freedom." With clinical experience, Dr. Sutton (who mostly treats children and adolescents) learned to avoid certain situations where she knows she might be attacked for her ideas, specifically her psychoanalytic ideas. When she was a student and a junior practitioner, she had less choice over which conferences she would attend and where she would present her work, which meant less of an ability to control encounters with practitioners who might critique her professional work or broader perspective. Her treatment often involves play therapy (a fundamental tool of psychologists who work with children), from which she can glean insight into a child's psyche. Dr. Sutton described encounters with practitioners who are unfriendly to psychoanalytic treatments:

Let's say I present a child case, how I work, and what I do. I have a strong theoretical base. But I use a lot of my clinical experience, so I work with metaphors. I work with play a lot, and when people ask me "do you have the proof of what you are doing?" I can explain, of course, but there are some limits about explaining the proof. You have to work with the imagination of people . . . then I can explain what is the symbolic functioning of playing and all that stuff. But there's always a limit [on proof]. "What you're doing is bullshit. You know? It doesn't make any sense. There is no immediate goal. You don't tell the child anything." No, I never tell a child what he has to change . . . so it's a very different clinical experience.

In describing her avoidance of conferences other than those hosted by the American Psychoanalytic Association, and practitioners who she sees as hostile toward her practice, Dr. Sutton is clear that tensions between psychoanalysis and biomedical psychiatry still exist and are palpable for Psychodynamic Psychologists. Further, Dr. Sutton highlights that the current emphasis placed on evidence-based medicine underlies the critiques and even hostility toward the dynamic model and the practitioners who employ it. Many of the Biodynamic Psychiatrists also report abstaining from mainstream psychiatry conferences, though it is much more about the identity issues I described earlier for them; they experience less contention as they are less likely to be singled out as different because of their medical training. Both the Biodynamic and Psychodynamic practitioners face tensions in encounters with Biomedical Psychiatrists, but it is a matter of degree; Psychodynamic practitioners are more likely to feel hostility and to have a sense that they are seen as lower in the hierarchy, although any psychoanalyst might be challenged for what is now more than ever before a fringe treatment paradigm.

A number of interviewees described these conflicts as having existed in psychoanalytic training as well.[5] For instance, Dr. Livingston explained,

I think there's tension on many levels: there's tensions at the institutional levels where still, even though we accept psychologists and social workers now, they're still kind of a minority. . . . I think they [the senior people in the field] still have a lot of skepticism about whether you can really do analytic work. I just had an experience—I gave a talk last weekend about [a psychodynamically informed treatment] at a conference for clinicians that also presented cognitive behavioral treatments and medication treatments, and during one of the breaks, a more senior woman came and said she was an analyst, and said she really appreciated my talk.[6] And then she mentioned something about the show on HBO called *In Treatment* where there's a therapist who's kind of psychodynamic but he's a psychologist and he doesn't seem to be doing classic psychoanalysis. He's doing some loose version of psychodynamic psychotherapy. And she made some kind of dismissive comment, "Oh, he's just a psychologist so that's why he's acting that way. And since we're analysts we wouldn't do that." It was like she didn't realize I was a psychologist, and I said, "Well, you know, you can be both." And she looked at me a little puzzled, like she hadn't reconciled those two things yet. So that's the kind of attitude you sometimes bump into with more senior people sometimes.

In Dr. Livingston's tone and her multiple uses of the word "sometimes," I sensed trepidation I'd felt from other Psychodynamic Psychologists in disclosing tense encounters with senior analysts. This is not surprising given the very people they're critiquing are in positions of power and may be current or former mentors. Dr. Haman described a similar experience in seminars during her psychoanalytic training: "There were discussions, not that many, but sometimes there would be discussions that would come up that would have a relevance for psychiatrists that would have a very different or nonrelevance for a psychologist. And it wasn't acknowledged that there was anybody in the room who didn't have medical training." This, they say, can make psychologists feel left out or even condescended to, and it happens both during and long after training. Though many of them feel that the starkest tensions between the psychiatrists and psychologists at their analytic institutes have dissipated (a few even say they do not exist anymore), there are clearly instances where psychiatrists, mostly unintentionally, complicate treatments or denigrate psychodynamic psychologists. Unlike Biodynamic Psychiatrists, Psychodynamic Psychologists experience tensions both from outside the psychoanalytic community as well as from within.

"I'm Cut from a Different Cloth"

Psychodynamic Psychologists often articulated a sense that they are unlike psychiatrists, and they largely attributed that difference to their graduate training. Consider the following response from Dr. Brighton when I asked for her thoughts about her psychiatrist colleagues' use of the DSM as the central diagnostic tool: "One type of training is trying to categorize, coming out of the medical model: what's the illness, what's the disease, what kind of pills are we gonna give them?

They have four years of training in those pills. That's heavy-duty training. That's what residency is. Psychologists are coming at it with who is the whole person? You can't quickly categorize that. And you wanna have a dynamic formulation, you wanna have an understanding of how this person has been put together. It's a different orientation." Dr. Brighton attributes the key differences between Psychodynamic Psychologists and psychiatrists to "heavy-duty" training in diagnosis and psychopharmacology. Psychiatrists, she indicated, have trouble getting away from the biomedical model. She explained, "It's their bible, but I think it can be extremely limiting, and what I see in teaching psychiatrists who are now psychoanalysts, it's very interesting to see them try to get out of their bible." Dr. Brighton teaches at her psychoanalytic institute, so she sees first-hand that psychiatrists struggle to be open to analytic ideas—to step outside their psychiatry lens that they acquired through training that focuses on diagnosis and treatment primarily using medication.

When Psychodynamic Psychologists and mainstream Biomedical Psychiatrists encounter one another, I was told it is sometimes as if they're speaking different languages. Though they have much more in common with Biodynamic Psychiatrists, Dr. Brighton told me she is increasingly aware of differences between her and her Biodynamic colleagues, as her career progresses. She noted, "More and more I see that I'm cut from a different cloth. I think many of us do . . . many of us feel different." As her expertise in psychoanalysis deepens with experience, and particularly when she encounters psychiatrists at the outset of their psychoanalytic training, she finds they exist in two different worlds; divergent primary professional socialization colors the remainder of their careers, even after psychoanalytic training. While the Psychodynamic Psychologists generally described the differences between themselves and Biomedical Psychiatrists in terms of conflict or exclusion, this was only occasionally the case with the Biodynamic Psychiatrists, with whom they typically seemed to assume that they shared greater similarities, given their psychoanalytic training.

Yet one of the clearest ways in which they set themselves apart from their Biodynamic colleagues was by alluding to their own strengths as analysts and talk therapists. Sometimes it seemed to become clear to them as we spoke how much richer their training in psychodynamic thinking was in graduate school, and my questioning about whether they feel different from a Biodynamic Psychiatrist allowed them to highlight their own expertise, a rare opportunity in a field that privileges a model in which they are not proficient. Psychodynamic Psychologists often pointed to their own training experiences as a way to highlight the difficulties their Biodynamic colleagues had as they transitioned into psychoanalytic training. Dr. Kent says of her experience in psychoanalytic training that it was "very continuous." "I'm not really doing something very different from what I did when I started graduate school," she explained. "It's different in that I know a lot more and I'm better at it, but it seems like the same kind of thing, whereas for them [the psychiatrists], it feels very discontinuous, and so they all seem like someone who in some way changed careers or something." If a psychiatrist were to have a largely psychoanalytic practice, it would indeed be like she changed careers, especially for the most junior Biodynamic Psychiatrists I spoke with, who were almost entirely trained in the biomedical model. The reality is that very few of the Biodynamic Psychiatrists practice much psychoanalysis at all once they complete their training, though they certainly do think more psychodynamically than their Biomedical Psychiatrist counterparts. Regardless, this notion that psychologists are better than the Biodynamic Psychiatrists at psychodynamic thinking, even before analytic training, was widespread.

Although some practitioners described psychoanalytic training as an equalizer of sorts—as Biological Psychiatrists become Biodynamic and acquire the skills to understand their patients more deeply—Psychodynamic Psychologists tended to describe a sense that core differences remain. A number of the Psychodynamic Psychologists struggled to say whether they think the differences between them and Biodynamic Psychiatrists dissipate by the time they are in the field practicing psychoanalysis. I heard uncertainty, for example, when Dr. Kent, who is several years beyond analytic training, told me the following:

> Psychologists tend to come to analytic training with much more experience . . . and a psychoanalytic point of view, whereas the MDs don't tend to. I think that really washes out over time, so that with colleagues that are my cohort now, I don't sense that it's that different. [She takes a long pause]. I'm sort of hesitating 'cause I'm not sure. I do feel like there's something about being an MD that feels different inside them, but I'm not sure quite how. I mean 'cause there's all kinds of funny slightly competitive issues.

Dr. Kent agrees that Psychodynamic Psychologists come into analytic training with talk therapy experience, which makes them quite different from Biodynamic practitioners, and although she was clear that psychoanalytic training makes her psychiatrist colleagues more like her, she also seemed certain that psychiatrists retain a somewhat enigmatic sense of difference, which she and others attribute to a combination of their primary professional socialization and selection in terms of who chooses to train in psychiatry in the first place. Dr. Brighton also explained that psychoanalysis brings different kinds of practitioners together, but the differences between psychologists and psychiatrists do not wash out. "I think we're trained very differently," she told me.

> The MDs and the PhDs are different kinds of people and have different kinds of training. PhDs are trained in philosophy and they are more broadly read in theory. It's a certain kind of person who comes to psychology and it's a different kind of person who becomes a doctor. What brings them together is psychoanalysis. Certainly, by the time they come into psychoanalytic training, they're both interested in the mind and the brain and analytic theory, but the kind of people, they think differently. I find that very interesting. I find that very stimulating. The doctors, the psychiatrists, tend to be very cut through the data, cut through the detail; they have wonderful memories, they gobble up articles in five minutes, the speed of learning is amazing, but the psychologists tend to be, they're better clinicians. They have a better grasp of—very often they have a less didactic and rigid—the medical model, something about the way the medical model trains psychiatrists with diagnosis and symptoms is a little bit antithetical. I mean, Freud said it's something antithetical to a philosophical grasp of the whole patient. And I think the psychologists get it by and large better.

There is a common notion among Psychodynamic Psychologists that they are more suited for the psychoanalytic training (though not necessarily that they are better at it after training) and of the psychiatrists as practitioners who struggle with psychodynamically oriented thinking, at least early on, largely because they are trained so heavily in diagnosis.

Unlike their descriptions of their psychiatrist counterparts, Psychodynamic Psychologists portray themselves as adept at psychodynamic thinking even before psychoanalytic training. For instance, Dr. Livingston explains,

> Because I went to a graduate school that was already so psychodynamic, I actually had learned a lot before . . . so in a way I felt like I started off a little bit ahead in terms of my theoretical knowledge, and to some degree my clinical experience because most of the psychiatrists who come in come in really right after residency or they've had maybe a couple longer term cases that lasted a little while or they had a supervisor who was psychodynamic, but other than that they don't really have that much knowledge and experience. So, it's funny 'cause you're starting off, in a weird way, ahead in terms of some of your knowledge, so it's kind of like comparing apples and oranges 'cause it's people who are at two stages of

learning. Now my experience in the course of the training, you know, they pick it up and they're very facile by the time [they finish] their training.

Dr. Livingston is also clear that primary professional training—medical school for the Biodynamic group and graduate school in psychology for the Psychodynamic group—results in practitioners with two different schemas for understanding and treating patients:

> So, in terms of attitude towards training, I wonder if psychologists are a little bit, because we're trained in psychology where, at least in my graduate school and I think in most, you're taught to be critical. You're taught to not take what's being taught to you at face value, but many professors encourage you—it's your job to critique these theories and come up with alternate theories and to test them and test their limits out and see what they can and can't explain. My sense is that physicians and psychiatrists don't always have that attitude toward theory. It's more received wisdom that—not always, but sometimes you get that sense that once they find kind of an approach that's aesthetically pleasing to them and they've had some success with presentations or that their supervisor or their analyst seems to be in accord with, it's kind of like they're locked in and that's it. I mean, this is a broad generalization, but I've sensed that before and it can happen with psychologists too, but I just sense a little bit more tendency to be openly critical, to challenge, to not accept at face value certain things, which actually I think makes over time for a little bit better clinical work because you don't get blinded by an etiological position and you can be a little bit more flexible with your patients.

Dr. Livingston explains that Psychodynamic Psychologists and Biodynamic Psychiatrists come to psychoanalytic training with very different organizational structures; she argues that whereas graduate training encourages students to question accepted knowledge, medical training encourages the memorization of models. In line with her colleagues, she says she thinks analysts from all training backgrounds have much more in common with each other after the analytic training. Yet the majority of the Psychodynamic Psychologists, like Dr. Willow, report a similar sentiment to Dr. Livingston about being better prepared than physicians for analytic training. She says, in talking to medical doctors, that they "tell me they have to unlearn more than psychologists, social workers, pastoral counselors, psychiatric nurses because they get trained 'you're the doctor and you are the authority.'" According to Dr. Willow, being a medical doctor makes Biodynamic Psychiatrists think of themselves as different from the Psychodynamic Psychologists, but it also makes it more challenging for them to assimilate dynamic principles into their approach to treatment.

A handful of Psychodynamic Psychologists felt that the tensions in the psychoanalytic community between psychologists and psychiatrists are no longer problematic precisely because since nonmedical practitioners have increasingly trained alongside medical doctors in psychoanalysis, psychiatrists have come to see their own shortcomings in in-depth treatments. Dr. Adams explained, "Psychiatrists have come to recognize that they have less therapy training when they come to psychoanalytic training than psychologists do, so I think a psychiatrist who's willing to go for psychoanalytic training already has to have a certain kind of humility because they're exposing themselves to psychologists and social workers who know much more about therapy than they do." Dr. Adams has a somewhat different perspective than many of her Psychodynamic colleagues; the notion that psychiatrists in analytic training are more humble than previous generations is not widely shared, though Dr. Adams points to a reality that only the psychiatrists who are the most open and interested in psychoanalysis would ever enroll in that type of training today, which means they are, in theory, less rigid from the start. Dr. Adams confirms her colleagues' assessment that psychologists have a deeper training in talk therapy that stems from their earlier exposure to it and their lack of exposure to training in psychopharmacology and minimal training in DSM diagnosis.

Living in a Biomedical World

While all the practitioners in this study live in a biomedical world, the consequences of practicing under its auspices vary based on (1) whether they are able to practice within the biomedical model, specifically by prescribing medications; (2) whether and to what extent they are trained to think medically and diagnostically; and (3) whether they are trained in psychodynamic ideas or psychoanalysis and how central it is to their practice. As the biomedical model has settled in as the dominant treatment modality in psychiatry, the greatest tensions exist for practitioners either who are not able to prescribe medications or who (generally because of exposure to psychoanalytic principles) are not entirely aligned with the biomedical model. While the majority of my interviewees agree that psychodynamic treatment can be useful, it has little relevance to the Biomedical Psychiatrists, especially as a chief treatment paradigm. As such, practicing in a biomedical world is relatively unproblematic—and generally advantageous— for Biomedical Psychiatrists. For Biodynamic Psychiatrists, training in analysis can cause interpersonal tensions, and because it is hard (maybe impossible) to truly integrate the models, they generally align themselves with one model or the other. In this way, some practitioners are still mired in the divisions that existed as the biomedical model rose to dominance. Luhrmann (2001, 5) describes the absolute separation between psychiatric camps in medical school classrooms in the 1990s: "Some mornings, men would come in wearing white medical coats. They would talk about neurotransmitters and catecholamines and draw diagrams of biochemical interactions on the board. . . . Other mornings, men . . . would arrive in tweed jackets, wearing spectacles. They would sit, hands folded, and talk with us about loss, mourning and the nadir point in psychotherapy." While the tweed jacket-wearers have become significantly less influential (and considerably more likely to be women), the division between the two models remains problematic for practitioners at the intersection of the two.

Along with the literal tensions embodied in interpersonal conflict and cognitive discord, these contradictions push practitioners to identify more closely with one paradigm over the other. Older analysts tend to think of themselves mostly as analysts, dropping the potential incongruities of practicing medicine, while junior Biodynamic Psychiatrists tend to feel more connected to their psychiatry training and often allow their psychoanalytic training to take a back seat. Psychodynamic principles inform their treatment, but they rarely practice any traditional analysis. Indicative of how times have changed is the extent to which the boundaries around psychoanalysis have become more porous than ever. Luhrmann (2001, 112) explains that psychodynamically oriented psychiatrists were unlikely to use diagnostic language when supervising residents—psychoanalysis remained largely cut off from biomedical psychiatry. This, however, is no longer the case. That Biodynamic Psychiatrists routinely talk about diagnosis, medication, and biological etiology is representative of the advanced state of the medicalization of psychiatry and of the ongoing role even psychoanalysts play in supporting the biomedical model (Smith 2014). While identifying more with psychoanalysis may cause tensions for the senior Biodynamic Psychiatrists, their junior colleagues are situated squarely in the biomedical model and identify as such.

For Psychodynamic Psychologists, not being able to prescribe medications and having no training in the biomedical model causes interpersonal clashes and ongoing reminders that they exist outside the mainstream of treatment and a feeling that they are lower in the hierarchy compared to Biodynamic Psychiatrists. These feelings are likely exacerbated by the various ways in which psychiatrists are treated as more valuable practitioners, particularly by insurance companies that reimburse their sessions at a higher rate than their psychologist counterparts and in hospitals where psychiatrists lead treatment teams. Psychodynamic Psychologists' experiences are reminiscent of early debates in

American psychoanalytic circles as to which practitioners have the right, and the best training, to practice psychoanalysis. Abbott (1988, 2) offers useful insight here into the importance of viewing the mental health fields, and psychiatry in particular, as a profession like any other: "A fundamental fact of professional life," he argues, is ". . . interprofessional competition. Control of knowledge and its application means dominating outsiders who attack that control. . . . Jurisdictional boundaries are perpetually in dispute, both in local practice and in national claims." Though the psychiatrists I spoke with (both Biomedical and Biodynamic) do not seem as actively engaged or invested in a fight for control as they once were now that the biomedical model is dominant in the field, the nonmedical practitioners describe a sense that psychiatrists seek to keep them on the outside or do not respect their way of thinking or their mode of practice as being equal. And in the way psychologists talk about their experiences in the field, there is a sense of being kept lower in the ranks.

Although practitioners in the mental health fields at large are relatively unaffiliated and even unaware of psychoanalysis as a treatment paradigm, being a psychoanalyst, within the psychoanalytic community and in the New York City mental health professions, is considered by some to be a badge of honor; it marks practitioners as highly trained talk therapists with skills few others in the United States have today. Furthermore, Psychodynamic Psychologists feel better suited for psychoanalysis than their Biodynamic colleagues. Yet the dominant treatment model in the field includes psychopharmacology, which requires introducing another practitioner into the treatment for a Psychodynamic Psychologist, who has no choice but to interact with practitioners who sometimes do not see psychoanalysis as an important or even legitimate treatment tool.

The extent to which practitioners experience these conflicts is rooted not only in whether they have medical credentials but also in how they were trained, who their mentors were, and what cohort they were a part of. Knowledge of and attitudes toward the biomedical model (everything from the centrality of diagnosis and medication to belief in biological etiology), talk therapy, and psychoanalysis vary principally based on how and when practitioners were trained. In short, living in a biomedical world for practitioners who believe deeply that psychopharmacology is the proper course of treatment is relatively uncomplicated and causes little tension. For psychoanalysts, the experience is different. The Biodynamic Psychiatrists point to the tensions between their two treatment approaches, but can largely avoid the fallout from the contradictions. Not only can they prescribe medications, but they have been trained to think diagnostically and largely adhere to a narrative of etiology that privileges biological

factors. The Psychodynamic Psychologists have much less agency and control
when it comes to eschewing these conflicts; in their view, their psychology training prepares them to be psychoanalysts better than any other discipline, yet
they lack the power and prestige that comes along with a medical degree. In
addition, they are much more likely to think about psychological and environmental causes of their patients' symptoms and to feel some skepticism about
the extent to which everything is biologically based. At the same time, Psychodynamic Psychologists have found ways to moderate their feelings of exclusion
or inferiority not only by referring their patients to trusted colleagues and practitioners they feel confident will share their psychodynamic interpretations of
patients' experiences and symptoms but also by pointing to their lack of psychiatry training as a boon—they are specialists in what they see as an effective
and therefore integral approach to treatment, in a way that medical professionals simply are not today.

The Dangling Conversation—Ambiguity in Mental Health Practice

In their 1966 hit song "The Dangling Conversation," Paul Simon and Art Garfunkel reflect on love lost. With allusions to art and literature, the narrator recalls he and his partner would "speak of things that matter with words that must be said." "Lost in the dangling conversation," the couple ponder existential matters and infamous questions like "can analysis be worthwhile?" and "is the theater really dead?" Though somewhat hyperbolic, the quotidian conversations of this likely educated, upper-middle-class duo in the late 1960s offers insight into the normative critique of psychoanalysis in popular culture even in its heyday. Discussion of the process, principles, and value of psychoanalysis was unremarkable not only in music, but also in film and literature, and was fervent within the mental health professions. Ongoing conversation (sometimes contentious) is endemic to a theory of the mind based on exploration and analysis—one that has gone through various stages of evolution, but withstood internal divisions for more than a century. Biomedical psychiatry has much less frequently been subjected to questions of its worth, and only dissenting voices have publicly raised concerns about its efficacy or the validity of its basic principles; for much of the late twentieth century and into the early twenty-first, psychiatry has operated under a biomedical paradigm, largely evading the kind of scrutiny that, although diminished, remains targeted toward psychoanalysis and psychodynamic psychotherapy. In this final chapter, I turn to a pervasive though often subtle sense of conflict and ambiguity around the various types of treatment my interviewees make use of. In particular, in practitioners' responses to my questions about the biomedical model, though many tended to support or even privilege it, there appears to be a burgeoning conversation about its fallibility, particularly the shortcomings of psychopharmacology and the problems with the myopic lens fostered by discrete diagnosis. And yet I saw little evidence of any immediate impact on practice, and although my interviewees suggested that change is possible, many of them are not sure precisely what kind of transformation they even hope for.

Among the psychoanalysts I spoke with, there remains a lively debate about the appropriate role for the psychodynamic approach in mental health treatment and how best to make use of its richness and depth. Having moved on from the era of psychodynamic dominance, practitioners who remain committed to psychodynamic practice still foreground the therapeutic relationship and exploration of patients' unconscious in their treatments. Yet as a freestanding treatment paradigm, psychoanalysis is on the periphery of psychiatry and most other mental health fields today. Even some of the psychoanalysts I spoke with do not always use the psychodynamic model as their primary mode of treatment. Along with medication, some use "supportive" and manualized treatments like cognitive behavioral or dialectical behavior therapies.

A range of structural constraints and cultural conditions relegate in-depth talking treatments to the sidelines of mainstream practice and traditional psychoanalytic treatments—and to some extent its practitioners—to marginal status. In the context of biomedicine, psychodynamic treatment is seldom employed, and there is sometimes a lack of clarity around what even counts as a psychodynamic or psychoanalytic treatment. As Schechter (2014) noted, psychoanalysts do not always agree on what counts as an analysis: Is it only the traditional four-times-per-week treatment where the patient lays on an analytic couch? Or can three-, two-, or even one-time-a-week treatment be considered psychoanalytic if the framework is sufficiently psychodynamic? My interviewees' perspectives on these matters varied, and there is avid debate among practitioners who consider themselves a part of the psychodynamic tradition about how to integrate psychodynamic principles into a successful practice in the current era. That my interviewees discussed these matters and participated in the lingering debate about the utility and unclear mechanism of psychoanalytic treatments was not surprising; it is in line with the dangling conversation that continues around psychodynamically informed treatments.

Despite this ongoing debate, as my interviewees describe it, the battle waged in hospitals and in the field more broadly in the 1980s and 1990s between advocates of biomedical treatments and those wedded to psychoanalysis has muted, and in most places is nonexistent today. The medicalization of the field has progressed to an advanced state, and the merits of psychoanalysis are largely an intellectual conversation among only those who practice it; it is considered a stand-alone treatment approach by only very few practitioners. Though I heard occasional stories of supervisors who still denigrate psychoanalysis or who think training in analysis is not worthwhile today, outside the small group of analysts, most practitioners are simply not concerned with it. In short, psychoanalysis presents no threat to the widespread practice of psychopharmacology or the dominance of biological thinking in the field. There are few remnants of the staunch divides most scholars noted in the late twentieth century between proverbial white-coat-clad diagnosticians and bearded, cigar-smoking analysts (see, e.g., Klitzman 1995; Luhrmann 2001).

It would likewise be no revelation to hear psychoanalysts express skepticism about the extent to which the biomedical model has taken over the field; there are significant consequences for practitioners whose primary treatment model is not in line with biomedicine and whose professional lives are complicated by the sidelining of psychodynamic principles from psychiatric treatment. What was unexpected was the sometimes subtle but pervasive sense of murkiness I encountered as practitioners attempted to explain etiology, and the efficacy and mechanism of the biomedical approach. And the majority of my interviewees, even the Biomedical Psychiatrists, expressed at least some concern about the overuse of psychopharmacological interventions and the myopia of the DSM. In the way my interviewees talk about their practice and their philosophies of thought and emotion, and particularly when they talked about how training has changed or the troubles facing current residents and interns today, I observed looks of concern. In such moments, my interviewees' tone often conveyed a sense of uneasiness, even anxiety, around the narrowly biomedical lens they feel junior practitioners come to see through before they even head out into practice. Despite the biomedical model's claims to having solved much of the uncertainty and lack of validity that the mental health field was lacking prior to the 1980s, there were prevalent if tacit references to a lingering ambiguity around the variety of psychiatric conditions my interviewees treat, even those they encounter most often—various types of depression, anxiety, and attentional problems. I also heard both blatant critiques and more subtle allusions to a tension between the widespread dominance of the biomedical approach and the less overwhelming evidence of its efficacy.

Pendulum Swings and Circuitous Paths

While all the practitioners I spoke with included biological factors and neurochemistry in their descriptions of etiology and treatment, the ubiquity and power of the biomedical model and its nearly forty years of settling in as the dominant mode of treatment seem to have given practitioners some space to see its fallibility, shortcomings, and inadequacies. In the late twentieth century, scientific inquiry, equated with objectivity, led to an increased call for proof of efficacy, and the complexity of psychoanalytic concepts simply did not lend themselves to being operationalized in quantifiable terms. Psychoanalysis was not, as its critics were known to point out, evidence based; among many other factors, this complexity, immeasurability, and opacity ushered in its demise as the key treatment modality. Biomedical psychiatry—armed with discrete diagnosis that claimed to increase validity and reliability, and psychopharmacology as its central tools—seemingly met this criterion, and managed care, pharmaceutical companies, and even patients quickly promoted the notion that the tools of the biomedical model ought to be the primary way of conceptualizing, identifying, and treating mental health troubles (Horwitz 2002a; Conrad 2005). Yet as some of my interviewees pointed out, the notion that the new psychiatry of the 1980s has demonstrated efficacy in the manner it intended to or that biological etiology is more than a theory is also open to debate. To be sure, psychoanalysts were more likely than their Biomedical Psychiatrist counterparts to express skepticism of psychopharmacology, but even those who regularly prescribe medications and who described etiology as largely biological sometimes alluded to uncertainty around the derivations of the conditions they treat and even of the efficacy of the medications they regularly prescribe.

Some of this ambiguity appeared in a lack of specificity in many of my interviewees' descriptions of etiology and the mechanism of psychopharmacological treatment. Even the most psychopharmacologically oriented practitioners offered largely taken-for-granted explanations about stabilizing neurochemicals or avoided talking about neurochemistry at all and instead focused their descriptions on the role of medication in treatment—on careful diagnosis and prescribing. At other times, I encountered forthright critiques of psychopharmacology or biomedicine more generally. While many of the practitioners I spoke with expressed optimism that more knowledge of the brain is on the horizon and that neuropsychiatry will at some future point be able to better tailor psychotropic medications to specific symptoms and specific patients, most practitioners also believe it may be unreasonable to expect this kind of psychopharmacological breakthrough anytime soon, if ever. And some practitioners indicated a lack of clarity around where they think the field is headed or where they think it ought to go.

There appears to be a somewhat behind-the-scenes (at times seemingly surreptitious) conversation about the shortcomings of the biomedical model. Within the context of these interviews, many practitioners pointed to uncertainties and conflicted feelings about the dominance of biomedicine. Biomedical

Psychiatrists were less likely to express these views, given their training and practice, but most at least alluded to insufficient evidence or complex, uncertain etiology. When it came to psychopharmacology, the more exposure practitioners had to psychodynamic principles, the more likely they seemed to evaluate it with some skepticism. Those who were more senior and had witnessed various treatment trends wax and wane were more apt to recognize that knowledge is fleeting and that theories are always in flux. Questioning the biomedical model seemed to feel much more natural to senior practitioners, particularly Biodynamic Psychiatrists like Dr. Gold, who is partial to the psychodynamic approach in her own work, but feels strongly that practitioners should have exposure to multiple models. No single paradigm, she explained, has all the answers. In the context of her critical assessment of psychopharmacology, I asked if Dr. Gold thought psychiatry was moving in a positive direction. She seemed to take issue with my use of the term "positive" and indicated that the field is not necessarily moving forward at all: "There's a play by George Bernard Shaw. I can't remember which one, but there's an old physician, and some issues come up and this guy says, 'Oh yeah, we had that idea fifty years ago.' I think the rest of medicine is moving progressively in their understanding of diseases. I'm not sure if psychiatry—I mean there's more understanding of biological substrate of schizophrenia and manic-depressive illness and so forth, so there is some progress going on, but not everything—is going in one direction. It's mixed." What is critiqued one moment and outmoded the next may return to prominence again, as did the biological model after its early twentieth-century demise. Dr. Gold's reference, I assume, is to *The Doctor's Dilemma*, an early 1900s play about medicine in pre–National Health Service Britain. Subtitled *A Tragedy*, the play acknowledges the inherent dilemmas of a medical profession in which doctors are influenced by financial gain and where medical intervention is preferred. Shaw's (1909) preface to the play is a broad-scale indictment of doctors and the medical profession. I can only assume that Dr. Gold's association to the play is not only because it reminds her that knowledge runs in cycles, but because it is apropos of many of the issues she believes still complicate the practice of medicine today. It was in this context and because of the disappointments with the medical model, particularly with psychopharmacology, and what she described as the "quick fix" model, that Dr. Gold told me the "pendulum" may be "swinging back" toward psychodynamic thinking. Dr. Gold also explained that psychiatry seems to suffer from more uncertainty than the "rest of medicine." While she feels other branches of medicine may indeed be moving forward, she was not sure if she would characterize psychiatry in the same manner. And for that reason, she feels optimistic that there may be a place for psychodynamic thinking in the gaps left behind, and because of the unful-filled promises of the biomedical model.

Still, a return to psychodynamic prominence seems unlikely. Some of the analysts in this study tend toward overgeneralization based on their own small group of colleagues in New York City, who are more influenced by psychody-namic thinking than most others in the United States today. Rumblings about a resurgence of psychodynamic thinking—more than a handful involving a pen-dulum analogy—are more likely here than anywhere else. Very few people expected the biomedical model to take over the field so quickly and so com-pletely in the 1980s; particularly older psychoanalysts still seem somewhat shocked at how relatively smoothly the biomedical model maintains its promi-nence despite its own shortcomings and unclear mechanism. They see room for a reintegration of psychodynamic ideas into the field. While their optimism about the future of psychodynamic treatments does not seem to realistically foreshadow a resurgence of psychoanalysis, it does seem to reflect a broader, burgeoning evaluation and even critique of the biomedical model. Some inter-viewees expressed a realization that, as Decker (2013, 319) notes, "antipathy to virtually all of psychoanalysis did not serve the psychiatric profession well and perpetuated the profession's harmful pattern of extreme swings between mate-rial and non-material forms of knowledge." These oscillations are natural and perhaps necessary moments in the evolution of the field, yet the tendency to revere one paradigm particularly at the expense of another is problematic, espe-cially, my interviewees point out, when the treatment brand of vogue is imper-fect and when the seemingly archaic method still has much to offer.

In recognizing that no one model can solve all problems, practitioners pointed to some of the shortcomings of the biomedical model. Dr. Taylor, one of the youngest and most junior of the Biodynamic Psychiatrists I spoke with, echoed Dr. Gold's prediction of a pendulum swing. She explained to me that, in what many referred to as the "post-Prozac era," there may be an openness to dynamic principles and practices, specifically to address the failings of psychopharmacology:

I would say that there has been a swing, you know, from a psychoana-lytic paradigm to a very biomedical paradigm that really kind of, I think, has gone past its peak, and that there is some recognition that not every-thing can be fixed with medications. This kind of initial optimism that medication would cure everything, kind of like what happened with psy-choanalysis in the fifties, psychoanalysis was gonna cure everything, a lot of excitement and then reality set in that well, it's good for some things but not for others. Same exact thing, I think, has happened with medication, so that while there's a lot of pressures to view things in a strictly medication, biomedical model—especially financial pressures, managed care, things like that—that there's something, kind of accumulated experience, the post-Prozac experience, that it doesn't do everything. And so I think there's a little bit more of a kind of a synthesis going on where people kind of accept that you kind of need more than one thing for a lot of people. Now what the other thing is—I think right now in the therapy aspect of it, that cognitive behavioral therapy is going through the same thing that psychoanalysis went through in the fifties, that Prozac went through. This is *the* treatment. If everybody just had cognitive behavioral therapy, everybody would be cured of everything, and I think that that's gonna go through the same thing, and ultimately, I think that the future is that we're gonna have a much more nuanced view of this.

Nuance, Dr. Taylor argues, is the goal; no single model can explain everything. Yet it is also clear from her description how entrenched the field is in biomedicine. She describes that various paradigms in psychiatry have been revered prematurely as magic bullets; as she and others indicated, the field is swayed by what some called "fads." It is clear, however, that Dr. Taylor takes for granted that the "synthesis" will consist of psychopharmacology and something else. The something else is unclear—is it psychodynamic psychotherapy, is it cognitive behavioral therapy, or is it a new treatment modality? She begins by recognizing that medicine can't solve all problems, but she closes by insinuating that "the other thing" is in addition to medication in a combined treatment—psychopharmacology is the static part of the treatment. Not a single practitioner suggested that psychopharmacology, despite its shortcomings and what they described as a kind of "overvaluation," would lose its role as a principal treatment modality. There was a tendency to recognize the potential role for talk therapy (even psychodynamic psychotherapy) precisely because of the shortcomings of the biomedical model and also remaining committed to the idea that psychopharmacology will endure as the central form of treatment in the field.

Because the etiological forces behind psychiatric symptoms remain vague, practitioners follow their training, generally believing that the model they were taught to employ is what's most beneficial for the patient in front of them. But they do so mostly in good faith. Practitioners sometimes struggle with the scant conclusive evidence in their field. Nearly forty years ago, Light (1980, 341) pointed to "garbled thinking which continues to plague the profession." He argued this leads to grasping at seeming certainty, and even to paradigmatic silos. Despite some new knowledge about the brain, much remains unknown. The degree to which my interviewees consider etiology to be fundamentally biological varies considerably, but the more they believe it, the simpler it was for them to explain both why their patients experience the kinds of symptoms they treat as well as how best to treat those problems. Yet I was surprised at the struggles many of my interviewees experienced in explaining the causes of their patients' symptoms. It is a difficult proposition to explain the amalgamation of the widely divergent entities seen as appropriate for psychiatric and psychological intervention, which leads to conflicts around how best to approach the treatment of the incredible range of emotions, experiences, and conditions mental health practitioners encounter; everything from trauma and grief to relationship troubles, delusions, and hallucinations are under their purview. Practitioners regularly noted that it was hard to describe etiology in part because, for example, a personality disorder is likely to elicit different ideas about etiology and treatment compared to substance abuse or a bipolar disorder. When I asked about etiology in regard to the conditions they treat, practitioners often seemed a bit overwhelmed and would ask me for a more specific question. Sometimes interviewees responded to my questions about etiology by talking about specific conditions, typically those they treat most commonly, like major depressive disorder or generalized anxiety disorder, as a way to narrow our conversation and make it feel more manageable. Other times they would speak in general terms about the impact of the environment or neurochemistry. It was also not always easy for practitioners to explain what the nitty-gritty work of their practice is. And in many of my conversations, especially with psychiatrists, there was a palpable tension between recognizing a lack of confirmatory evidence and maintaining a sincere belief that biology and neurochemistry underlie the kinds of problems their patients experience. Even the majority of psychoanalysts, who have extensive training in clinical theory, are not always expert at explaining what it is that they do. They often explain how psychoanalysis works by resorting to broad or vague explanations of transference or the unconscious. Psychiatrists often have more seemingly straightforward explanations when they speak, for example, of the impact of antidepressants on specific neurotransmitters. As I have described throughout the book, both explanations are somewhat murky, but psychoanalysts have learned to speak with less certainty and authority (and also have more nuanced explanations that are in line with psychodynamic thinking), while psychiatrists speak with the support of biomedicine behind them and about theories of etiology and treatment that are in line with the currently dominant thinking. This provides an impression of clarity and concrete knowledge that was much less likely to appear in psychoanalysts' conversations about, for example, the connection between trauma and current symptoms or between conflicted thoughts and symptoms. In short, despite the ambiguity around all models, psychopharmacology and biomedical explanations seem more concrete.

The DSM and Murkiness

A key tool of evidence-based medicine, the DSM is largely responsible for this somewhat illusory comfort—a sense of greater certainty than is possible. Many of the practitioners I spoke with recognize that they are acting on positivist notions that they can identify and treat their patients' conditions as discrete entities. Even the most biomedical of my interviewees typically pointed out the impossibility of narrow categorizations of human thought and emotion (even if in addition to praising its ability to organize thinking). Grob and Horwitz (2010, 163) likewise emphasize the false sense of validity the DSM provides. In their discussion of major depressive disorder, the most commonly diagnosed mental illness in the United States today, they argue,

> The DSM has generated a consensus about the operational definition of depressive disorder. It has not, however, resolved any of the issues about classification that have continuously surrounded the condition since the earliest times. Whether depression is continuous or categorical, how many categories it has, what its relationship to melancholic personality is, and how it can be distinguished from normal sadness are no closer to resolution now than they were when the DSM-III arose. . . . "Are we still confused?" asks an article written in 2008. It responds, "The answer is surely 'yes.' Our current nosologies remain as 'working hypotheses.'"

Yet confusion has not detracted from the adherence to DSM categories, one function of which is to make it possible for practitioners to see the problems they treat as clear-cut entities, which Fujimura (1987) argues makes action seem more straightforward and tasks more doable. The DSM, representative of formal disease classification in psychiatry, is an icon of the current school of thought, which Light (1980) described as an "ideological resolution of uncertainty." Medicine's inherent uncertainty (Fox 1997) is precisely what makes evidence-based medicine so appealing to doctors, especially to psychiatrists, who do not have the same objective measures as those in, for example, cardiology or oncology. Cassell (2004, 214) similarly surmised that the focus on disease at the expense of other elements of personhood or the context of patients' lives aids practition-ers in "denying the inevitability of uncertainty." At the same time, Cassell describes one of the central achievements of becoming a seasoned physician as the ability to work within and around uncertainty (Cassell 2004), an inherent contradiction in the practice of medicine.

When my interviewees spoke about the central role of the DSM in mental health treatment, their conflicted feelings came to the fore. Discrete diagnostic categories, in Conrad and Schneider's (1992) terms, represent both a "bright" and "dark" consequence of medicalization. Practitioners readily described the major gains and perils associated with symptom classification, yet recall that most of my interviewees laughed off the centrality of the DSM to their practice or talked about how other people—but not they—use it too rigidly. Often in the same breath, they reported its significance in the field, but indicated that DSM diagnoses represent only a starting point to treatment. Many report using the DSM because they feel stuck between a rock and a hard place. On one hand, they see DSM-like categorization as offering greater reliability in diagnosis (the lack of which is precisely what led to the fall of the psychodynamic model). They are also often required by insurance companies or practice guidelines to provide DSM diagnoses. On the other hand, they describe that more creative diagnosis and assessment of patients, getting away from DSM categories, dem-onstrates an ability to think in a nuanced manner and typically marks practi-tioners as entering a more advanced career stage. And they note that overly rigid categorization is not an accurate snapshot of patients' experiences and emotions anyway. The trouble is that the DSM, as a number of my interviewees explained, represents the knowledge in the field and extensive collaboration of clinicians and researchers. And when my interviewees describe why they use the DSM and why they often rely on biomedical understandings of etiology and biomedi-cal interventions, it is clearly not just because of their association with evidence-based medicine or because of pressure to fall in line; it is also because the structure of such a diagnostic endeavor allows practitioners to overlook or at least avoid the unknowns associated with the biomedical model.

In their descriptions of the troubles with the advanced state of medicaliza-tion in psychiatry, practitioners focused mostly on dilemmas they've encoun-tered with the DSM, and many called for a less discrete system of diagnosis and increased scrutiny in the prescribing process. Especially when psychiatrists spoke of current residents and trainees, I was often told that less rigidity in adhering to the biomedical model and more openness to alternative perspec-tives would solve some of the problems practitioners find most troubling, but this is also in direct opposition to the claims of gains in validity via the use of the diagnostic model. These kinds of conflicts around the DSM not only were common in practitioners' narratives but also were rarely expressly identified or discussed. As I described in detail in chapter 3, one of practitioners' greatest concerns with overly rigid diagnosis pertains to residents and other junior practitioners, who, their more seasoned colleagues worry, are less equipped to attend to the experience of illness and eschew deep knowledge of their patients in favor of focusing on seemingly recognizable symptomatology. Largely outside psychiatry, scholars have raised similar concerns (Cassell 2004; Horwitz 2002a; McWilliams 2000; Smith 2011), and though very few psychiatrists have publicly expressed such worries, my interviewees' responses suggest that they are clearly present. In the context of describing his training experiences, Klitzman (1995), for example, noted the tendency for the biomedical model to drive practitioners toward diagnosis and away from meaning and contextualization. Compared with Biomedical Psychiatrists, Biodynamic interviewees more pointedly noted a loss from both the absence of psychodynamic principles and the narrow focus on diagnosis and psychopharmacology for their residents and other trainees; and as all my interviewees described the potential pitfalls for junior practitioners, they got to the heart of many of the larger issues they deem crucial for the field more generally.

Lamenting the Loss of Psychodynamic Ideas

In addition to their conflicted feelings around the DSM, most practitioners described their residents' and interns' lack of exposure to alternative models, and specifically to psychodynamic ideas, as a point of concern about the future of the field, which offers further insight into the conflict they feel around the monopoly biomedicine and a diagnostic, evidence-based model more generally have on training. Practitioners in all three groups regularly told me that interns' and residents' lack of exposure to thinking beyond diagnosis and psychopharmacology is troubling. Some trainees, especially in New York, may happen into a mentorship or training program where psychodynamic principles are valued, but most do not. And if they do not, the odds of ever being exposed enough to consider training further or of even learning the most basic psychodynamic principles are slim. Hale (1995, 340) pointed to drastically increased odds of patients choosing analytically oriented therapy if they are a "friend and supporter of psychotherapy," and the same is true of medical practitioners. Especially for psychiatrists, if they didn't have a family member or close other who exposed them to psychodynamic principles or they didn't encounter psychodynamic ideas early in their training, they were likely to make diagnosis and psychopharmacology their primary if not only mode of treatment. This is reminiscent of

Strauss and colleagues' (1981, 369) suggestion that "while a number of institutional conditions may affect professional fate . . . interaction with other ideology-bearing professionals is critical." "For the advancement of most professionals," they argue, "other professionals are the critical publics." Many Psychodynamic Psychologists also noted a similar trend in their field wherein psychodynamic principles are much less present than ever before in training programs; interns are much more likely to become familiar with cognitive behavioral and other short-term, manualized treatments.

Even those who manage to gain exposure to the psychodynamic approach know that to train well as a psychodynamic psychotherapist (especially as an analyst) would involve significant time, labor, and money, which may not feel worthwhile. Further, the perceived efficacy and efficiency of psychopharmacological treatments for psychiatrists and of behavioral treatments for psychologists make psychodynamic psychotherapy seem like a much more complex and less certain intervention by comparison. And building and maintaining a practice around psychodynamic treatment is a difficult task; several Biomedical Psychiatrists told me they couldn't imagine financially sustaining that kind of practice. This is a reality that the continued practice of psychoanalysis is up against—one that has significant consequences for the type of treatment practitioners are likely to offer, and consequently patients are likely to receive.

Despite these various forces driving the field toward the biomedical model, many of my psychiatrist interviewees do feel a sense of loss that their field has become so focused on psychopharmacology. In noting the forces that have driven psychiatrists to practice less talk therapy, Eric Plakun, chair of the American Psychiatric Association's committee on psychotherapy by psychiatrists, noted a decade ago, "It really is a loss to our patients if they aren't getting psychotherapy. . . . Psychiatrists are in a unique position to provide psychotherapy because they really have the medical training that allows them to integrate medication and therapy, mind and body" (Kaplan 2008, 8). Plakun and many other psychiatrists, many of my interviewees included, see themselves as integrators along these lines; however, because of their ability to prescribe medications, but given the current structural and cultural forces at play, which typically lead to little exposure to psychodynamic training, it is unlikely that residents are offered the full array of tools.

The lack of psychodynamic training in psychiatry and its relative absence from practice also reflects an increasing uncertainty over who should perform which elements of mental health practice. Should psychiatrists practice psychopharmacology exclusively, as has increasingly been the case? Or should these biomedically trained practitioners retain some of the skills (even the most basic) of psychodynamic psychotherapy? There are a range of structural and cultural impediments to the latter including an ever-increasing division of labor and complexity in both the field of mental health and medicine at large. The goals of biomedical treatment and psychodynamic psychotherapy and psychoanalysis are different in some key ways, and the practice of psychoanalysis is not in line with psychiatric or broader culture, which largely support efficient intervention and the alleviation of clearly identified symptoms in measurable ways. Light (1980, 340) noted nearly forty years ago that one of the reasons practitioners were drawn to biomedical psychiatry and psychopharmacology is that it seems like an antidote to the confusion in the field around what role psychiatry in particular ought to play: "Psychiatry today seems as confused about how to train its members about their roles relative to physicians, paraprofessionals, and nonmedical therapists as ever. The confusion is less obvious, because spokesmen keep uttering to each other reassuring phrases about 'medical psychiatry' . . . viewing the profession as a whole reveals confusion and unresolved questions around the classic fault lines in the profession." What I heard from nearly all my interviewees was an acceptance of the biomedical model (with some pushback mostly from Psychodynamic Psychologists) and a great deal of "reassuring phrases about 'medical psychiatry'" (in terms of both its efficacy and its dominant role in the field) from nearly all the psychiatrists and some psychologists. Despite the critiques of psychopharmacology, all the psychiatrists I spoke with (save the handful of older Biodynamic Psychiatrists) tended to describe medications and the biomedical model as the most effective, especially for severe symptoms, and to feel responsible for offering biomedical solutions given their biomedical training. The Psychodynamic Psychologists were also quick to recommend psychopharmacology referrals when patients presented with severe symptoms. The uncertainty about biomedicine is typically hidden behind an outward allegiance to and promotion of the biomedical model, which contributes to the continued, largely exclusive training in the biomedical model.

My interviewees claimed that it's important to integrate various treatment models, and the term "eclectic" was batted about regularly in our conversations about treatment approaches, yet the primacy of the biomedical model has required little in the way of adaptation from most Psychiatrists including those I call Biomedical. The advanced state of biomedical psychiatry typically means others must adjust to the biomedical model and a health care system that relies on discrete diagnosis and broadly favors psychopharmacological intervention. Psychoanalysts and other psychodynamically oriented practitioners have largely been the group to adapt and find ways to work with and around the biomedical model (Decker 2013). McWilliams (2005, 148) explains,

> On the simple ground that they help people, I expect that the traditional psychotherapies, and the values they honor, will survive. But they may do so only outside the health care mainstream. In response to insurance-driven limits on treatment, some professionals have already redefined what they do as "coaching," an activity that can be marketed to those who can pay out of pocket. Other therapists simply reduce their fees for less wealthy patients who need more comprehensive, personalized treatment than their health plan offers (though there is a limit to how generous clinicians can be without becoming self-defeating). We all find ways to adapt, to keep doing what we value, whatever the social context. Whether therapeutic values can enter public discourse and influence how mental health questions are viewed nationally, however, remains to be seen.

The last four decades have involved significant modifications to practice by nonmedical practitioners like McWilliams, and a period of relatively little challenge for psychiatrists trained in biomedicine.

An Unclear Future

The practitioners in this study indicated an emergent recognition of the fallibility of the biomedical model; they conveyed signs of a nascent conversation about the underlying uncertainty around psychopharmacology and biological etiology. Yet the biomedical monopoly over psychiatric thinking and practice remains relatively unmoved; some argue it has only become enhanced as new biomedical technologies and interventions are increasingly available. Even though there is a growing realization that antidepressants in particular are not the magic bullets they were thought to be just two decades ago, I saw little evidence that the Biomedical Psychiatrists, particularly the most junior of them, who were trained fairly strictly in the DSM model and psychopharmacology, are particularly interested in integrating in-depth talk therapy into their practice. They may see a role for it in the field, but they do not seem to see themselves as paradigmatic integrators. Even among the psychiatrists I interviewed, many of whom told me they had exposure to psychodynamic ideas because they practice (and many trained) in or near New York City, there is little tangible movement away from the biomedical model. Furthermore, many of my interviewees for whom the psychodynamic model is important were clear that outside their circles, the principles of psychodynamic psychotherapy rarely if ever even enter the conversation around etiology or treatment.

Regardless of whether some interviewees believe in the efficacy of or even hope for a pendulum swing back toward intensive talking treatments, I did not see evidence for this trend represented in practice. Most practitioners, even those who do not think of themselves as active proponents of the biomedical model, are at the very least passively supporting its dominance. And while even the strict psychopharmacologists described the merits of using multiple models—some in fact prided themselves on using various tools in their treatment approach, in line with the biopsychosocial model that they told me characterized their training—they privilege a biomedical approach and largely attribute their patients' symptoms to genetics and other biological factors. Though there are exceptions, the influence of the psychodynamic model on the Biomedical Psychiatrists I spoke with seems largely to consist of a consideration of some immediate life context and a recognition that doctor-patient relationships matter, whereas the practitioners who trained in psychoanalysis used terms like "depth" and "transference" to describe their treatments. In other words, saying one is in favor of an eclectic treatment model or that one values the use of talk therapy does not necessarily reflect any impact on practice.

There is very little active resistance to the biomedical model, and as such, clinicians uphold the medicalization of a range of conditions from everyday troubles to severe conditions (Smith 2014). This is perhaps most clear in looking at practice composition. Of the thirty psychoanalysts, only ten had as many as four active psychoanalytic cases at the time I interviewed them; the average was four patients in analysis for Biodynamic Psychiatrists and two for Psychodynamic Psychologists (many analysts consider their three-times-per-week patients as being in analytic treatments). Still others who are trained as analysts do not see any analytic patients; a lot of the younger Biodynamic Psychiatrists told me they trained in analysis to be better therapists, but none said they necessarily wanted to have analytic practices. To be clear, all the Psychodynamic Psychologists and most of the Biodynamic Psychiatrists also had significant numbers of patients in less intensive talk therapy—patients they typically see twice a week. It is difficult to sustain a traditional psychoanalytic practice, even for my interviewees whose patients often pay out of pocket. While none of my interviewees had practices composed entirely of psychoanalytic patients, psychodynamic psychotherapy retains a significant role in many of my interviewees' practices; Biodynamic and Psychodynamic practitioners are deeply connected to psychodynamic principles and believe that many of the conditions they treat can be ameliorated using these principles, even outside psychoanalytic treatments.

Whether or not practitioners were exposed to even the most basic psycho-dynamic principles in training has a clear impact on practice. The Biomedical Psychiatrists who had been exposed to psychodynamically trained mentors offered perhaps the most obvious insight; these psychiatrists were much more likely to tell me the guiding principles of psychoanalysis shape their work, even in short-term, medication-based treatments—they may think about patients' early lives, wishes, and conflicts, even if they don't design a treatment based on those factors. In this regard, there is support for Metzl's (2003) argument that the biomedical model has not entirely replaced the basic principles of psycho-dynamic treatment, like transference. Yet it seems clear that the more psycho-pharmacologically oriented a practitioner is, the less the chance there is that she has developed any meaningful expertise in the application of basic psycho-dynamic principles. And even when Biomedical Psychiatrists did describe an interest in psychodynamic ideas, they were unlikely to apply them in their prac-tice; there is a stark contrast between applying dynamic principles while con-ducting a largely medically oriented practice and treating patients in intensive psychotherapy. Perhaps one of the clearest obstacles to applying psychodynamic principles while under the influence of the biomedical model is that the most basic principle, the relationship between the practitioner and patient, is diffi-cult to develop and nearly impossible to use as a central part of the treatment given short and infrequent sessions that characterize mental health treatment today.

Though the biomedical model has offered great relief to patients (and some-times to practitioners) and brought a sense of clarity and scientificity to the field, and though it tends to be the default for many of my interviewees, most of them were clear that no one treatment can do all the heavy lifting. Further, most practitioners (though not all) acknowledged some uncertainty around etiol-ogy and treatment as well as a desire for trainees, whether psychiatry residents or psychology interns, to have exposure to multiple models. Seeing much of human behavior and emotion as in need of intervention and feeling driven to solve problems biomedically are somewhat in tension with the recognition that the biomedical model can't solve all problems. I want to end by saying that over-all, while some of them never mentioned it directly, my interviewees' narratives (sometimes their own words and wishes for the field) demonstrate the impor-tance of maintaining psychodynamic principles at least in the background.

At the outset of this book, I described an awkward interaction I had with Dr. King (Biodynamic) at her suggestion that I should "go to medical school and become a psychiatrist." I proposed that the central reason for her comment (and similar statements by other doctors) was that the biomedical model is the default for thinking about issues around mental health; perhaps it did not quite make sense to her that sociology would be an appropriate lens for investigating the kinds of subjects I described as central to this project. Dr. King's comment also represents a resistance to thinking in ways outside the biomedical model, which sometimes seemed palpable in conversations with a good number of my interviewees, particularly those who were medically trained. While she tended to default to the biomedical model especially when our conversation turned to symptoms that meet criteria for DSM diagnosis, or that, in her mind, cause too much suffering, Dr. King is an analyst and she was quick to point out the importance of patients' conflicted thinking and interpersonal relationships and the significance of in-depth talk therapy. Given her psychoanalytic training, Dr. King was not as rigid in her biomedical thinking as, for example, Dr. Sutter (Biomedical), whose portrait appeared in chapter 2, and who does not have any psychodynamic training or any theoretical or treatment model outside her biomedical training.

While psychoanalysis is unlikely to be an option beyond its current population of practitioners and patients for a range of reasons, the principles of psychodynamic psychotherapy could be more integrated into mainstream psychiatry. One potential avenue for doing so is via the continued development of interventions that integrate psychodynamic principles into shorter-term, manualized treatments that are accessible to a wider range of patients and practitioners than traditional psychodynamic psychotherapy or psychoanalysis. This would have consequences for practitioners' and patients' experiences alike. For example, Panic Focused Psychodynamic Psychotherapy (PFP), Transference-focused Psychotherapy (TFP), and Regulation Focused Psychotherapy (RFP; for children) all offer the potential to bring psychodynamic principles into an evidence-based model. My interviewees suggested that analysts are also working on other creative ways of offering their treatments to wider audiences, but the increasing division of labor between psychiatrists and other mental health practitioners along with issues around reimbursement further complicates the feasibility of such an endeavor. Furthermore, because of the structural and cultural forces that maintain its dominance, the biomedical model as a paradigm—as a way of thinking about etiology, treatment, and broader issues in terms of the goals of the mental health treatment—is even more resistant to change than the psychodynamic model was in the mid-twentieth century. For this range of reasons, the biomedical model seems not to be going anywhere anytime soon. Despite the questions my interviewees raised about the biomedical model, and even though there is a great deal of uncertainty around the kinds of symptoms their patients present with and the future of their own field—to a greater or lesser extent depending on their training and practice—the psychiatrists in particular not only tended to accept the dominance of the medical model but also both overtly and more tacitly suggested that it is the right way to think about people and help with their troubles.

How might today's practitioners in training—interns and residents in a range of mental health professions—acquire the kinds of skills most of my interviewees suggested they lack, and many suggest they would benefit from? While some residency programs, recognizing the dearth of training in psychodynamic ideas, have instituted seminars or limited course work in a range of talk therapies, and some have even assigned texts critical of the biomedical model that push young practitioners to think beyond discrete diagnosis, there is little opportunity to engage with models beyond the biomedical. What might it look like to offer practitioners the chance to more richly and deeply explore these ideas that they might employ in their practices to fill the gaps in strictly psychopharmacological or cognitive behavioral approaches? How might it strengthen the field for practitioners—those with no intention of becoming analysts or even psychodynamic talk therapists for that matter—to have adequate training in the basic principles needed to enrich their treatments beyond medication management? Though many Biodynamic Psychiatrists endeavored to train in psychoanalysis with the hopes of having a more traditional talk therapy practice, a significant number trained in psychoanalysis simply to be better therapists and to acquire the tools of the psychodynamic approach, even if it is ultimately not their main treatment tool. And they did so because there really was no other avenue for them to learn these skills given the current state of psychiatry training.

From the early until the late twentieth century, psychodynamic thinking was in the proverbial foreground of psychiatric and other mental health practice and figured prominently in the American cultural landscape, while the biological thinking that had dominated the field in pre-Freudian days remained in the shadows. Over the course of the late twentieth century, the biomedical model came into focus in mental health treatment, as it did in American culture at large for thinking about and treating a range of physical and emotional troubles. The biomedical model solidified its place as the salient treatment paradigm in psychiatry, relegating psychoanalysis and psychodynamic psychotherapy to the fuzzy, out-of-focus background, and then into obscurity by the turn of the twenty-first century. The psychodynamic model is now almost undiscernible. But my interviewees suggested that, while psychoanalysis and psychodynamic treatments are not likely to ever be in the foreground again, the most basic principles could come back into focus just enough to remain apparent—they might just linger in the background for practitioners who would benefit from, for example, thinking through the meaning of the relationship they have with patients and how early experiences may shape current functioning and symptomatology. If greater numbers of practitioners had some psychodynamic training, the use of psychodynamic psychotherapy and psychoanalysis might expand beyond populations with the greatest financial resources and cultural capital, something the majority of my psychoanalyst (and some Biomedical) interviewees seemed to wish for. The narrow focus of the biomedical model, particularly on diagnosis and psychopharmacology, obscures the range of human thought and emotion the majority of my interviewees describe as essential to an understanding of the symptoms their patients typically experience. This limited perspective is also one reason social scientists have much to offer with continued study of the role practitioners play in upholding the biomedical model and the consequences associated with the advanced state of medicalization.

Notes on the Method and Sample

This project is based on forty-three semistructured interviews with psychoanalysts and psychiatrists whom I recruited using an initial convenience sample, and then a snowball approach. All interviewees practice in the New York City area, although they were trained at various hospitals and graduate programs around the country, and in three cases outside the United States. I carried out interviews in practitioners' offices, with the exception of four that took place in interviewees' homes, when practitioners simply could not fit the interview into their work schedule and were kind enough to offer me their leisure time. Interviews typically lasted forty-five minutes, as I designed them to fit into one standard talk therapy session, hoping not to upset practitioners' schedules or cost them a more considerable wage loss. This worked well for practitioners who are primarily talk therapists, but those who practice mostly psychopharmacology often see two or even three patients for medication management visits in that time, so this interview proved to be a bigger imposition on them than I had anticipated. On occasion, I had to adapt to a thirty-minute time frame for psychopharmacologists, which was largely unproblematic as fewer of my queries about talk therapy were applicable to them. Their conversational style also tended to be more concise compared to practitioners trained in psychoanalysis.

Interviews were semistructured, and wherever possible I let my interviewees guide the conversations, though I had a number of structured questions and I was typically able to cover all of them even if indirectly. Interviews focused on three substantive areas: (1) professional background, including training, major shifts in the field, and thoughts about psychiatric/psychoanalytic practice in general; (2) practice and treatment preferences, including thoughts about etiology, and why patients enter treatment; and (3) theoretical and philosophical questions including opinions about what suffering is and how it should be conceptualized as well as the rise of new disorders and new DSM categories.

I digitally recorded all interviews for accuracy, with the exception of one interview with a Biomedical Psychiatrist who declined at the advice of her counsel. I took extensive notes during her and all other interviews and added summary notes about my impressions immediately after interviews. I transcribed the verbatim text of the interviews within forty-eight hours following each interview. I excluded direct quotes from the one aforementioned interviewee, as I cannot be sure they are entirely precise. I proofread all transcripts multiple times, and two of my students also reread them for accuracy. I coded and analyzed all transcripts first by hand and later using Dedoose, a cloud-based data analysis software package.

I conducted the first forty interviews between August 2007 and May 2011. I added an additional three interviews with Biomedical Psychiatrists in September 2013 for two reasons: First, I recruited my initial interviews through some of the most psychodynamically oriented practitioners and wanted to add additional practitioners whom I was referred to by the practitioners with more psychopharmacological practices. I did so in order to ensure that I had a range of psychiatrists in my sample, and that I was adequately capturing the sentiments of psychopharmacologists. Second, I wanted to check that the release of

Table A1. Training and Practice Characteristics

Group	Degree/ Certification	Training	Typical Practice
Biodynamic Psychiatrists (n = 20)	MD/certificate in psychoanalysis	4 years of medical school, 1 year of internship in psychiatry, 3 years of residency in psychiatry, 5 years of psychoanalytic training	Psychopharmacology, psychodynamic psychotherapy, psychoanalysis
Psychodynamic Psychologists (n = 10)	PhD/certificate in psychoanalysis	4 (or more) years of graduate school, 1 year of internship, 5 years of psychoanalytic training	Psychodynamic psychotherapy, psychoanalysis
Biomedical Psychiatrists (n = 13)	MD	4 years of medical school, 1 year of internship in psychiatry, 3 years of residency in psychiatry	Psychopharmacology, infrequent talk therapy

DSM-5 had not had any significant impacts on the practices of the psychiatrists who use it most readily. I was quickly able to discern that there were not any significant differences between these newer interviewees and the original group.

Table A1 offers a quick reference to the training and practice characteristics that led me to categorize my interviewees into three distinct groups, and table A2 is an alphabetized master list of the practitioners in each group, even those whose words are not quoted directly in the text. Twenty interviewees were psychoanalytically trained psychiatrists who first attended medical school and completed residencies in psychiatry. Later they enrolled in psycho-analytic training programs, which required an additional five years of education in psychoanalytic theory and practice. To obtain a postdoctoral certificate in psychoanalysis, practitioners must also take on three analytic cases that are supervised by a training analyst and participate in approximately five years of psychoanalytic treatment with a different training analyst. Because of their dual training in both the biomedical and psychodynamic models, I dub these practitioners "Biodynamic Psychiatrists."

Ten interviewees were with psychoanalytically trained psychologists, who were trained in clinical psychology—their graduate training earned them a PhD

Table A2. Practitioners by Group

Biodynamic Psychiatrists	Psychodynamic Psychologists	Biomedical Psychiatrists
Dr. Brown	Dr. Adams	Dr. Brooks
Dr. Carroll	Dr. Brighton	Dr. Clarendon
Dr. Dean	Dr. Butler	Dr. Doughty
Dr. Elliot	Dr. Coffrey	Dr. Elm
Dr. Ferris	Dr. Haman	Dr. Evans
Dr. Gold	Dr. Kane	Dr. Hart
Dr. Halsey	Dr. Kent	Dr. Lawrence
Dr. King	Dr. Livingston	Dr. Morris
Dr. Lewis	Dr. Porter	Dr. Poplar
Dr. Linden	Dr. Sutton	Dr. Reeve
Dr. Madison		Dr. Stanley
Dr. Mill		Dr. Sutter
Dr. Nelson		Dr. Troy
Dr. Park		
Dr. Plymouth		
Dr. Remsen		
Dr. Sterling		
Dr. Sullivan		
Dr. Taylor		
Dr. Warren		

(rather than an MD). Following graduate school in psychology, they also trained in psychoanalysis (same process as above for the Biodynamic Psychiatrists). I call these practitioners "Psychodynamic Psychologists," since their training is almost entirely in the psychodynamic model in both their doctoral and post-doctoral training. Psychologists are not licensed to prescribe medications. Psychodynamic Psychologists provide an important comparison to the medically trained psychiatrists. They allow for insight into the extent to which medical training (especially in the current biomedical era) affects psychoanalytic thinking and practice. Furthermore, psychologists perform a great deal of the talk therapy practiced today, as psychiatrists have become increasingly trained as psychopharmacologists.

My final group is composed of thirteen psychiatrists, whom I call "Biomedical Psychiatrists" because their practice largely pertains to diagnosis and psychopharmacology; they do not have any formal psychoanalytic training, and most had very limited exposure to psychodynamic principles at all. There were two practitioners who were exceptions and had significant training in psychodynamic ideas, but they were not trained as psychoanalysts and only a few others were exposed to some of its basic principles in medical school. All the Biomedical Psychiatrists have practices where they see a significant number of patients for medication prescriptions only. Their practices range from pure psychopharmacology to those with some talk therapy patients (usually no more than once-per-week sessions and generally more focused on supportive treatments).[1] While some of my interviewees and some scholars have referred to this kind of practitioner—those who practice largely within the biomedical model—as Biological Psychiatrists, I feel Biomedical to be a more apt term for the practitioners I interviewed since they not only believe in biological etiology but also practice using key tools of the medical model: diagnosis and psychotropic medications. For additional description of the training process for all three groups, see chapter 2—"Practitioner Portraits and Pathways to Practice."

A few of my interviewees still work part-time in hospital settings, but all are in private practice, and with the exception of two, private practice takes up the majority of their working hours. Even if treating people only in outpatient settings, most maintain affiliations with hospitals through their involvement in teaching and mentoring. With the exception of one Biomedical Psychiatrist, my interviewees are not insurance providers. While they do often fill out insurance reimbursement forms, and sometimes have to deal directly with insurance companies to substantiate their patients' requests for reimbursements, the majority of their patients pay out of pocket; when insurance compensates for some of the treatment, patients are responsible for submitting claims. As such, compared to the general population of practitioners in the United States, the practitioners in my sample have more control over their practices. That they are not direct providers means my interviewees' patient pool is wealthy; my interviewees' patients are largely upper-middle and upper class, a fact most of the doctors in my sample are keenly aware sets their patients apart from the average Americans seeking treatment and them from the average practitioners providing it. My interviewees predominantly treat patients experiencing major depressive disorder or other forms of depression, anxiety, ADHD, and substance abuse problems. The psychoanalysts also specialize in treating troubles related to personality: narcissism, borderline personality, and so on. Some also specialize in treating patients who experienced various forms of trauma. Therefore, their ideas about treatment are also influenced by the kinds of illnesses and the type of population they are likely to see. Some of these practitioners do see patients with psychotic conditions or severe borderline personality disorder, which is notoriously difficult to treat, but this is not the common story for the private practice doctor.

Confidentiality

One of the most difficult parts of this project is the tension between wanting to protect practitioners' identities and representing the nuance and intrigue of our conversations. Some of the most interesting interchanges I had with practitioners were those around particular patients. My interviewees offered fascinating examples of their thinking and treatment decisions, much of which I cannot share in this book to protect both their confidentiality and that of their patients. As such, I have done my best to represent their thinking and treatment approaches, although there are many cases where I am not able to offer the reader as much evidence or insight as I would have liked. Interviewees' names in the text are all pseudonyms that I randomly assigned, and I do not describe any of the practitioners in depth; even in the four portraits, I have been careful to remove potentially identifying markers, opinions, training experiences, and affiliations. I typically identify practitioners only by whether they are Biodynamic, Psychodynamic, or Biomedical. For example, practitioners' ages ranged from thirty-seven to eighty, with an average of fifty-three, and age does drive their opinions, but I provide ages in the text only when relevant. In some cases I have also interchanged their practice locations or other descriptions of their personal appearances or that of their offices with other similarly trained practitioners. Given the small community, particularly of psychoanalysts, in New York

City, and given the snowball sample, it was important to decrease the odds of their identification by other interviewees they may have referred me to, by other colleagues or friends in the field, and by patients.

Perhaps most obvious is that I use the generic "she" throughout the book. Because the majority of my interviewees were women (twenty seven) and because gender is not of central importance in this analysis, the generic "she" offers another layer of confidentiality, and does not detract from the analysis of my interviewees' statements. The only way gender seemed to overtly shape the issues I discuss in this book was when psychiatrists described their choice to go into psychiatry over another field in medicine. Family obligations or the desire to have children made psychiatry feel a more reasonable choice for some of the women given gendered family expectations than, say, surgery (although some men mentioned lifestyle choices as well). That there were fewer men in the sample is probably a result of my having started with women contacts, who referred me to their friends first, who it seemed were more likely to also be women. Furthermore, one of my initial contacts specialized in child treatment, and therefore my snowball sample is skewed toward those who specialize in child and adolescent treatment (though these practitioners all treat adults as well). According to The Association of Medical Colleges' data, 53 percent of pediatric/child/adolescent psychiatrists were women in 2017, and although medicine at large remains male-dominated, psychiatry is one of the fields with an overall significant percentage of women practitioners. In psychology, there are far greater numbers of women than men in the field in general. In 2013, the American Psychological Association reported that there were more than two women psychologists for every man.

Uniqueness of the Sample

My sample dramatically overestimates the extent to which psychodynamic principles are valued and used in practice compared to the nation at large and should not be taken as a commentary on general trends in psychiatry or the mental health fields. However, because my interviewees are overall more wedded to psychodynamic treatment than the average American practitioner, they are an ideal barometer for examining the extent to which the biomedical model dominates the field. In other words, thirty of my interviewees, as psychoanalysts, are more likely to think psychodynamically of almost any practitioners in their field today. The way they think about the biomedical model likely underestimates its pervasiveness in the field at large, but is a very good threshold for understanding the extent to which medication and diagnosis are central to the field, and why in-depth talk therapy is kept on the periphery. In addition, my interviewees' practices are all in New York City proper or the surrounding suburbs, and all are in private practice, so their opinions about the field must be seen in that context, which is highly divergent from, for example, in-patient hospital psychiatry, in-network providers' practices, and practices in other parts of the country where psychoanalysis is rarely taught or practiced. It is also of note because of my snowball sample, the majority of my psychoanalyst interviewees trained at the same institute, and although all the psychoanalysts in this sample trained in and around New York City, psychoanalytic institutes vary in terms of their attitudes on a range of key issues, including who can train in analysis, what an analytic practice ought to look like, and even the basic guiding theories candidates learn.

Reflexivity

While I spent only a short period of time with each of these practitioners, who I am—or who practitioners imagined me to be—undoubtedly impacted the kind of information they shared with (or kept from) me, as is clear from the interchange I describe at the outset of this book with Dr. King. My presence is likely familiar to practitioners in a number of potential ways. With Dr. King and others, my interests allowed for projections of her own career pathway onto mine. As a junior scholar interested in the field of mental health, I was a potential practitioner, although in reality, medicine is entirely outside the realm of my academic strengths and career interests. As an academic, a woman, and someone familiar with the field, I am also the right demographic to be a patient, who is the usual visitor to their offices. I quite literally sat where their patients sit. In some cases, I was also the same or close in age to practitioners' children, which undoubtedly impacted how they heard and responded to my questions. Some interviewees were also aware that my mother is a psychoanalyst. To be sure, who I imagined them to be also impacted my analysis of their words. As a sociologist who is also the child of a psychoanalyst, I have come to know the mental health profession as a Simmelian stranger; I am neither completely foreign nor truly a member of the group. This basic position is likely what made this project possible at all and helped me to be able to identify many of the ambiguities and nuances of this world of mental health practice, but it pushed me as I analyzed the data to always keep in mind my own insider/outsider status.

Acknowledgments

When I was young, on my way to school or on juvenile forays around New York City, I often noted the shingles and nameplates of mental health practitioners that adorned the front yards, lobby entryways, and somewhat hidden side entrances of buildings, mostly in the city's affluent neighborhoods. These symbols of the ubiquity of mental health treatment were simply mundane background to me then. By the time I was in college, I was fascinated with the idea that, behind closed doors, there is a nearly constant stream of patients discussing their lives with professionals trained and employed to listen to their narratives and to offer various types of assistance to their often-painful symptoms. Of course, some of this curiosity came when my own mother began to use part of our home as her first private practice office. In graduate school, fully recognizing my own interests in mental health, I discovered that private practice mental health professionals are not often directly consulted and are rarely interviewed in studies on the mental health fields. Because of the nature of their work, its content is known relatively exclusively by practitioners themselves and their patients; practitioners are often not even aware of what their colleagues' practices look like. Furthermore, their schedules are typically filled with sessions, teaching, supervisions, and sometimes research, so it is not surprising that only rarely have researchers, even with access, ventured into the world of private practice. So, whenever they could see me, I crisscrossed the New York City area, from my home in Brooklyn to the Upper East Side, from Tribeca to the Upper West Side, from Midtown to Westchester County, from one waiting room to the next.

Being a researcher in a patient's world never felt entirely ordinary. The typical dynamic turned on its head, I sat in leather recliners and on couches meant for patients and interviewed practitioners, which was an unusual experience for me and I suspect for my interviewees as well. And yet I was welcomed, offered tea, coffee, and water, and on more than one occasion to partake in a home-packed lunch, as it became clear that my interviewees often graciously offered me their only free "hour" of the day. The practitioners who participated in this study invited me into their offices, their clinics, and even their homes on several occasions. Although much of what my interviewees do professionally is confidential, they often play significant roles in patients' lives—and have impacts that are largely unseen by the public, and even by those closest to their patients. While I have examined their words critically, I want to be clear that the desire to use their training to alleviate pain and suffering and to help patients lead more productive and fulfilling lives was always their primary goal. I am now more than ever before certain that it is important to study mental health practice from the ground up in order to avoid the mistake of overlooking the people who do this difficult but meaningful work—but people who are also fallible, and part of a larger system of paradigms and practices that are sometimes murky and less than fully substantiated. Practitioners often do the mostly unknown labor of implementing treatment approaches that further the knowledge in the field, and of interpreting research that doesn't always have clear clinical implications, and they journey along with patients as they experience the benefits and perils of those interventions. For sharing their thoughts and their often overbooked and valuable time, as well as their ideas about a profession and practice that is for most of them also part of a larger worldview, I am grateful to my interviewees. It was an enlightening experience to learn more about private practice, as I hope it will be for readers, and I hope this book makes clear why their voices are necessary in any conversation about the mental health fields.

Though I didn't entirely realize it then, my initial academic curiosity about mental health practice developed when I discovered the sociology of mental health during my undergraduate days in Janet Shope's seminar at Goucher College; that course helped shape my professional trajectory. It was also at Goucher that Jamie Mullaney helped me design my first interview-based project, which gave me the early tools I needed to uncover much of what is fascinating in practitioners' narratives, and where, nearly twenty years ago, Joan Burton taught me what it means to have a sociological imagination. I will forever be grateful to these three wise women for sharing their knowledge, and for their friendship and support over many years.

This project evolved over more than a decade, during which time Allan Horwitz and Debby Carr provided invaluable feedback on countless drafts, and offered more general counsel, all of which has shaped my thinking in innumerable ways, and for which I am continually grateful. I want to thank Phaedra Daipha for her ongoing guidance and friendship, and for the many hours she and Pat Carr spent with me once upon a time analyzing these narratives. I'm deeply thankful for my dear colleagues Christine Mair, Bambi Chapin, and Jennifer Hemler for their thoughtful feedback at various points throughout this process, for their support through research and life triumphs and woes, and for the many discussions that helped me press on, especially in moments of frustration. I'm lucky that Dawne Mouzon and I discovered mutual intellectual interests many years ago, which fostered not only a cherished friendship but also the chance to work on new areas that were an important respite from the solitary work of book writing. I'm also appreciative of the many days of writing companionship and camaraderie with Jamie Trevitt, Loren Henderson, for writing retreats with Kylie Parrotta, and for long-ago coffee shop days with Janet Lorenzen and Kate Burrows. And to all the friends and family who have been supportive during this lengthy process, especially Mileah Kromer and Laura Sicari, I am lucky to have you.

I am also thankful for kind and encouraging staff and faculty in my department at UMBC. I want to acknowledge two former students, Lila Scott and Brenda Kissane, who assisted many years ago with proofreading transcripts, as well as the team at Rutgers University Press, for strengthening this project at every stage, especially their reviewers for the valuable feedback that has improved both the structure and content of this book. I was also fortunate to be granted summer research funds for several years as faculty at both Goucher and UMBC, as well as resources from the Dean's Research Funds through the College of Arts, Humanities, and Social Sciences at UMBC, all of which aided in the completion of this project. The Eminent Scholar Mentorship program at UMBC also supported my concurrent research on other projects, and allowed for my continued work with Marta Elliott, from whom I have learned a great deal.

Kyle, thank you for your constant analysis of words, which encouraged me to choose mine carefully, although I suspect you'll have more to say about that. And to Michael, thank you for being my buddy, for traipsing around Manhattan with me on one crisp afternoon while I finished up the last round of interviews, for your silly sense of humor, and your years-long efforts at tiptoeing around our creaky, centenarian house.

Notes

Introduction

1. I refer to the current model in psychiatry as the "biomedical" model throughout the text as it encapsulates biological thinking about both etiology and psychopharmacology, as well as diagnosis, which is a central feature of medical practice more generally. Neither the term "biological" nor "medical" alone adequately captures the theoretical and practical approach my interviewees describe.

2. Also known as CBT, cognitive behavioral therapy is a short-term, less than twenty-week, manualized program wherein therapists work with patients on restructuring the way they think in order to change their behavior, with the goal of alleviating anxiety and other symptoms. It is highly active, involves routine exercises and homework assignments on the part of patients, and is considered to be evidence-based. An offshoot of CBT, dialectical behavior therapy (DBT), is another increasingly common model developed to treat patients with borderline personality disorder, but is now used for patients with depression and a range of other diagnoses.

3. This decrease in the use of talk therapy is less dramatic for patients who pay out of pocket, patients with diagnosed personality disorders and low-level depression, and patients seeking treatment in the northeastern United States. African Americans, Hispanics, people younger than twenty-five, and those with public insurance (such as Medicaid) are less likely to receive psychotherapy. Further, managed care tends not to cover more than a handful of talk therapy sessions, if any, but will usually cover short visits for medication management (Mojtabai and Olfson 2008).

1. From Meaning Making to Medicalization

1. Other psychological theories, such as Gestalt psychology and self-psychology (a form of psychoanalysis), had an impact on the field in the 1960s and 1970s. Most of these therapies developed in opposition to certain psychodynamic principles and were never as broadly impactful.

2. For a detailed description of pre-Freudian, asylum-era psychiatry, see Dowdall (1996), Grob (1994), Horwitz (2002a), Lunbeck (1994), Scull (2015), Shorter (1998), and Whitaker (2002).

3. The most succinct definition of neurosis can be found in "neurotic conflict," wherein instinctual drives are unable to be discharged. Tensions arise and "ego becomes progressively less able to cope with the mounting tensions and is ultimately overwhelmed. The involuntary discharges manifest themselves clinically as the symptoms of psychoneurosis. . . . Neurotic conflict is an unconscious conflict between an id impulse seeking discharge and an ego defense warding off the impulse's direct discharge or access to consciousness" (Greenson 1995, 17).

4. Though Freud was much more interested in the psychological underpinnings of neurosis, he firmly believed that there were biological roots to thinking and behavior—a drive toward outcomes. Sullivan (along with other prominent psychodynamic theorists of the time: Erich Fromm, Karen Horney, Clara Thompson, and Frieda Fromm-Reichmann) is responsible for the most notorious reworkings of drive theory, which he claimed was an inadequate explanation for neurotic behavior.

5. Especially later in his career, Sullivan's critique of Kraepelin became more pointed. He accused Kraepelin of mistaking symptoms of schizophrenia for behavior that stems from hospitalization; in other words, Sullivan claimed that rather than identifying anything truly characteristic of a certain type of illness, the Kraepelinian system risked inaccurately capturing behavior borne of the institutional environment, in much the same way as the antipsychiatry movement led by figures like Thomas Szasz would several decades later.

6. Neurotic conditions are those that are less severe such as anxiety, whereas psychotic conditions involve the most severe symptoms such as the delusions and hallucinations that characterize schizophrenia.

7. Deinstitutionalization describes the mass exodus of the mostly severely ill individuals into community settings. The intention was to shrink the size of the mental health care system, which was extremely costly and had been extensively criticized during the antipsychiatry movement (driven by Thomas Szasz in the United States and Michel Foucault in France) and the more general civil rights movements of the 1960s. It is considered to be one of the worst policy failures in American history, largely because deinstitutionalization ironically made the mental health field larger and more costly (Light 1980, 9) and because the community programs that were meant to offer support never operated in the manner intended (see Estroff 1981).

8. The basic ideas for DSM-III were based on diagnostic categories that came to be known as the Feighner criteria and were developed by a group of psychiatrists often referred to as neo-Kraepelinians because of their reliance on a strict classificatory system for the symptoms of mental illness. For a more thorough discussion of the development of DSM-III, see especially Hale (1995), Horwitz (2002a), Klerman (1977), Shorter (1998, 300–301), and Decker (2013).

9. The extent to which physical illnesses are as observable as evidence-based medicine suggests is itself questionable (Grob and Horwitz 2010).

10. Even earlier, new antipsychotic medications were also marketed and came to be seen as relatively safe and effective treatments for more severe illness, and this was thought to allow formerly institutionalized patients to live in community settings (Estroff 1981; Shorter 1998).

11. The brain scanning technologies included CAT (computed axial tomography), PET (positron emission tomography), and MRI (magnetic resonance imaging).

12. In the mental health professions at large, there is more fervent debate, usually involving psychologists, social workers, and other non–medically trained practitioners, though they too are highly influenced by clinical practice guidelines and managed care practices.

13. This lawsuit was filed in 1985 by a group of psychologists who wanted to train in psychoanalytic institutes run by the American Psychoanalytic Association, which maintained that only medical doctors were qualified to practice psychoanalysis.

14. Though the terms "psychodynamic" and "psychoanalytic" are used somewhat interchangeably, the key distinction is at the level of practice. While there is not a difference between the two in terms of the theory they represent, psychoanalytic practice describes classic treatment, three to five times per week, whereas even a sporadic treatment can be psychodynamically informed, which simply means it is influenced by core psychodynamic principles.

15. Psychology has also embraced evidence-based medicine and biological thinking.

16. It is difficult to accurately assess the number of practicing psychoanalysts in the United States. Consider the following comparison: while there are thousands of new

psychiatry MDs and psychology PhDs awarded each year, only a handful (about ten) of those graduates will enter each of the few psychoanalytic training programs in the United States each year.

17. There are a number of psychoanalytic training programs that have reputations for being the friendliest to nonmedical practitioners and admit greater numbers of psychologists and social workers and other practitioners than psychiatrists.

18. ICD (International Classification of Diseases) is the World Health Organization's measurement of illness around the world.

2. Practitioner Portraits and Pathways to Practice

1. See the appendix for a more complete discussion of the methodology. See specifically table A1 for a description of practitioners' training trajectories. See table A2 for a reference list of which practitioners were trained in which treatment approaches.

2. Later in our conversation, Dr. Nelson described cognitive behavioral therapy (CBT) as an example of these other evidence-based treatments. CBT is a short-term, no more than twenty-week program of therapy that focuses on changing thoughts and behaviors. Therapists and patients work with standard protocols including worksheets and homework assignments. It is generally used for anxiety, though versions of it have been adapted for other conditions as well.

3. The Promise of "Imperfect Communication" and the "Prison" of Rigid Categorization

1. In DSM-IV-TR, Axis I were considered clinical disorders, which include affective disorders like anxiety and depression. Axis II were personality disorders and intellectual disabilities (though the latter usually is not what practitioners are referring to; they use Axis II as a shorthand for personality disorders). When my interviewees refer to the two axes, they generally mean to make a comparison between mood (Axis I) and personality (Axis II).

2. My interviewees described using NOS (not otherwise specified) categories when a specific diagnosis (e.g., major depressive disorder) was not necessary or when they could not neatly fit a patient into a specific DSM category. See Whooley (2010) for other uses of the NOS category. DSM-5 eliminated the NOS category.

3. "Ticking off five out of nines" is a reference to checklists that use DSM symptoms as the basis of diagnosis.

4. Neurosis is a central concept in psychoanalytic theory. As I described in chapter 1, Freud distinguished between neurotic and psychotic conditions. The former are less severe (a normal part of life), while the later include severe symptoms such as delusions and hallucinations. Dr. Park's use of neurosis here is as a synonym for dynamic principles rather than the classic definition.

4. Etiological Considerations and the Tools of the Trade

1. Practitioners generally used the term "supportive therapy" to refer to talk therapy that is not geared toward deep exploration of the psyche, but rather aimed at helping patients cope with life troubles, improving general well-being and self-reliance. The relationship with the therapist is still important, but focused much more on empathy and support than on analysis.

2. According to the American Psychoanalytic Association (2009b), "Transference describes the tendency for a person to base some of her perceptions and expectations in present day relationships on his or her earlier attachments, especially to parents,

siblings, and significant others. Because of transference we do not see others entirely objectively, but rather 'transfer' onto them qualities of other important figures our earlier life."

3. According to the American Psychoanalytic Association (2009a), countertransference ". . . refers to the analyst's feelings and attitudes towards the patient: his/her reaction to the patient's transference, how his/her own experiences impact his/her understanding of the patient, and the analyst's emotional responses to the patient." Countertransference was thought by Freud to be an impediment to treatment, though today, when used properly in a treatment, it is generally thought to be a useful avenue for the therapist as clues to her own as well as the patient's personality and style of relating to others.

4. Compliance refers to patients' adherence to a treatment plan (e.g., taking prescribed medications as directed).

5. The Consequences of the Biomedical Model for Practice and Practitioners

1. This is very much a product of my sample, which is composed of clinicians in private practice in and around New York City. They are more exposed to psychodynamic ideas in training and through colleagues than is the case for clinicians elsewhere in the country, even if they do not officially train in it.

2. Another structural factor that tends to push practitioners toward the biomedical model is that psychiatrists who trained in the biomedical era (even if they are psychoanalysts) have the credentials and training to prescribe medication, and so some of their referrals are sent to them because they are psychopharmacologists rather than because they are psychoanalysts. This may change if they come to be known as good analysts by their colleagues and are then referred analytic patients, but that takes many years of developing an expertise and a reputation. Furthermore, it is more lucrative to see multiple psychopharmacology patients in an hour than one analytic patient.

3. This is a reference to the accusations of Biomedical Psychiatrists that psychoanalysts were narrow-minded and too quick to ignore the benefits of medications, perhaps to the detriment of their patients (see McWilliams 2000).

4. Though almost all of my Biodynamic interviewees do have some patients whom they see for medications alone, it is a much more common practice in mainstream psychiatry where practitioners' entire practices often revolve around diagnosis and medication.

5. This is likely less true in analytic programs where there are fewer psychiatrists; the majority of my interviewees trained in programs where psychiatrists had a significant presence. In fact, I was told that many psychologists choose programs with greater numbers of psychologists or social workers precisely to avoid tensions with psychiatrists.

6. Transference-focused psychotherapy (TFP) is a psychodynamically informed, highly structured treatment for borderline and other personality disorders.

Appendix

1. For this analysis I have purposely excluded social workers and other licensed mental health practitioners from the sample, as their training is different from that of psychologists and psychiatrists who undergo approximately the same number of years of training prior to psychoanalytic treatment. Other mental health professionals are also still excluded from clinical training in the American Psychoanalytic Association's institutes and therefore would not make for a fair comparison.

References

Abbott, Andrew. 1988. *The System of Professions: An Essay on the Division of Labor*. Chicago: University of Chicago Press.

Abraham, John. 2010. "Pharmaceuticalization of Society in Context: Theoretical, Empirical, and Health Dimensions." *Sociology* 44(4):603–622.

American Psychiatric Association [APA]. 1968. *Diagnostic and Statistical Manual of Mental Disorders*. 2nd ed. Washington, DC: American Psychiatric Association.

———. 1980. *Diagnostic and Statistical Manual of Mental Disorders*. 3rd ed. Washington, DC: American Psychiatric Association.

———. 1987. *Diagnostic and Statistical Manual of Mental Disorders*. 3rd ed., revised. Washington, DC: American Psychiatric Association.

———. 1994. *Diagnostic and Statistical Manual of Mental Disorders*. 4th ed. Washington, DC: American Psychiatric Association.

———. 2000. *Diagnostic and Statistical Manual of Mental Disorders*. 4th ed., text revision. Arlington, VA: American Psychiatric Association.

———. 2013. *Diagnostic and Statistical Manual of Mental Disorders*. 5th ed. Washington, DC: American Psychiatric Association.

American Psychoanalytic Association. 2009a. "Psychoanalytic Terms and Concepts Defined." http://www.apsa.org/content/psychoanalytic-terms-concepts-defined.

———. 2009b. "Theory and Approaches." http://www.apsa.org/content/psychoanalytic-theory-approaches.

Association of American Medical Colleges. 2017. "Active Physicians by Sex and Specialty." https://www.aamc.org/data/workforce/reports/492560/1-3-chart.html.

Barlow, David H. 1996. "Health Care Policy, Psychotherapy Research, and the Future of Psychotherapy." *American Psychologist* 51:1050–1058.

Bowker, Geoffrey C., and Susan Leigh Star. 2000. *Sorting Things Out: Classification and Its Consequences*. Cambridge, MA: MIT Press.

Brenner, Charles. 1974. *An Elementary Textbook of Psychoanalysis*. New York: Anchor Books.

Busch, Fredric N., Barbara L. Milrod, and Larry S. Sandberg. 2009. "A Study Demonstrating Efficacy of a Psychoanalytic Psychotherapy for Panic Disorder: Implications for Psychoanalytic Research, Theory, and Practice." *Journal of the American Psychoanalytic Association* 57:131–148.

Busfield, Joan. 2006. "Pills, Power, People: Sociological Understandings of the Pharmaceutical Industry." *Sociology* 40:297–314.

———. 2010. "'A Pill for Every Ill': Explaining the Expansion in Medicinal Use." *Social Science and Medicine* 70:934–941.

Cassell, Eric J. 2004. *The Nature of Suffering and the Goals of Modern Medicine*. Oxford: Oxford University Press.

Clarke, Adele E., Janet K. Shim, Laura Mamo, Jennifer Ruth Fosket, and Jennifer R. Fishman. 2003. "Biomedicalization: Technoscientific Transformations of Health, Illness, and U.S. Biomedicine." *American Sociological Review* 68(2):161–194.

Conrad, Peter. 1992. "Medicalization and Social Control." *Annual Review of Sociology* 18:209–232.

———. 2005. "The Shifting Engines of Medicalization." *Journal of Health and Social Behavior* 46(1):3–14.

———. 2007. *The Medicalization of Society: On Disorders*. Baltimore: Johns Hopkins University Press.

Conrad, Peter, and Joseph W. Schneider. 1992. *Deviance and Medicalization: From Badness to Sickness*. Philadelphia: Temple University Press.

Cuijpers, Pim, Annemieke van Straten, Lisanne Warmerdam, and Gerhard Andersson. 2009. "Psychotherapy versus the Combination of Psychotherapy and Pharmacotherapy in the Treatment of Depression: A Meta-analysis." *Depression and Anxiety* 26(3): 279–288.

Decker, Hanna S. 2013. *The Making of DSM-III: A Diagnostic Manual's Conquest of American Psychiatry*. New York: Oxford University Press.

Dowdall, George. 1996. *The Eclipse of the State Mental Hospital: Policy, Stigma, and Organization*. Albany: State University of New York Press.

Estroff, Sue E. 1981. *Making It Crazy: An Ethnography of Psychiatric Clients in an American Community*. Berkeley: University of California Press.

Falck, Hans S. 1980. "Aspects of the Sociology of Psychiatry." *Journal of Society and Social Welfare* 231:219–235.

Fleck, Ludwik. [1935] 1979. *Genesis and Development of a Scientific Fact*. Chicago: University of Chicago Press.

Fonagy, Peter. 2003. "Psychoanalysis Today." *World Psychiatry* 2(2):73–80.

Fox, Renee. 1997. *Experiment Perilous: Physicians and Patients Facing the Unknown*. Piscataway, NJ: Transaction.

Freidson, Eliot. [1970] 2007. *Professional Dominance: The Social Structure of Medical Care*. New Brunswick, NJ: Transaction.

Freud, Sigmund. [1940] 2003. *The Wolfman and Other Cases*. New York: Penguin.

Furedi, Frank. 2004. *Therapy Culture: Cultivating Vulnerability in an Uncertain Age*. New York: Routledge.

Fujimura, Joan H. 1987. "Constructing 'Do-Able' Problems in Cancer Research: Articulating Alignment." *Social Studies of Science* 17:257–293.

Gerrity, Martha S., Jo Anne L. Earp, Robert F. DeVellis, and Donald W. Light. 1992. "Uncertainty and Professional Work: Perceptions of Physicians in Clinical Source." *American Journal of Sociology* 97(4):1022–1051.

Gieryn, Thomas F. 1983. "Boundary-Work and the Demarcation of Science from Nonscience: Strains and Interests in Professional Ideologies of Scientists." *American Sociological Review* 48:781–795.

Gilman, Sander. 1987. "The Struggles of Psychiatry with Psychoanalysis: Who Won?" *Critical Inquiry* 13:293–313.

Graf, Elizabeth, Barbara Milrod, and Andrew Aronson. 2010. "Panic-Focused Psychodynamic Psychotherapy: A Manualized, Psychoanalytic Approach to Panic Disorder." In *Off the Couch: Contemporary Psychoanalytic Applications*, edited by Alexandra Lemma and Matthew Patrick, 160–175. New York: Routledge/Taylor & Francis.

Greenberg, Jay R., and Stephen A. Mitchell. 1983. *Object Relations in Psychoanalytic Theory*. Cambridge, MA: Harvard University Press.

Greene, Jeremy A. 2007. *Prescribing by Numbers: Drugs, and the Definition of Disease*. Baltimore: Johns Hopkins University Press.

Greenson, Ralph R. 1995. *The Technique and Practice of Psychoanalysis*. Madison, WI: International Universities Press.

Grob, Gerald N. 1994. *The Mad among Us: The History of the Care of America's Mentally Ill.* Cambridge, MA: Harvard University Press.

Grob, Gerald N., and Allan Horwitz. 2010. *Diagnosis, Therapy, and Evidence: Conundrums in Modern American Medicine.* New Brunswick, NJ: Rutgers University Press.

Hale, Nathan. 1995. *The Rise and Crisis of Psychoanalysis in the United States: Freud and the Americans, 1917–1985.* New York: Oxford University Press.

Healy, David. 2004. *Let Them Eat Prozac: The Unhealthy Relationship between the Pharmaceutical Industry and Depression.* New York: New York University Press.

Horwitz, Allan V. 2002a. *Creating Mental Illness.* Chicago: University of Chicago Press.

———. 2002b. "The Measurement of Mental Health Outcomes: Where Have We Been and Where Are We Going?" *Journal of Health and Social Behavior* 43:143–151.

Horwitz, Allan V., and Jerome C. Wakefield. 2007. *The Loss of Sadness: How Psychiatry Transformed Normal Sorrow into Depressive Disorder.* Oxford: Oxford University Press.

Hunt, Morton. 1993. *The Story of Psychology.* New York: Doubleday.

Hyman, Steven E., and Eric J. Nestler. 2005. *The Molecular Foundations of Psychiatry.* Washington, DC: American Psychiatric Press.

Jutel, Annemarie. 2011. *Putting a Name to It: Diagnosis in Contemporary Society.* Baltimore: Johns Hopkins University Press.

Kalinkowitz, Bernard N., and Lewis Aron. 1998. "Postdoctoral Program in Psychotherapy and Psychoanalysis: History of the Program." http://postdocpsychoanalytic.as.nyu .edu/object/pd.history.

Kaplan, Arlene. 2008. "The Decline of Psychotherapy." *Psychiatric Times* 25(13):1–8.

Karp, David A. 1996. *Speaking of Sadness: Depression, Disconnection, and the Meanings of Illness.* Oxford: Oxford University Press.

Kirk, Stuart A., and Herb Kutchins. 1992. *The Selling of DSM: The Rhetoric of Science in Psychiatry.* New York: Hawthorne.

Kleinman, Arthur. 1988. *The Illness Narratives: Suffering, Healing, and the Human Condition.* New York: Basic Books.

Klerman, Gerald. 1977. "Mental Illness, the Medical Model, and Psychiatry." *Journal of Medical Philosophy* 2:220–243.

Klitzman, Robert. 1995. *In a House of Dreams and Glass: Becoming a Psychiatrist.* New York: Simon & Schuster.

Kohler, Robert E. 1982. *From Medical Chemistry to Biochemistry: The Making of a Biomedical Discipline.* Cambridge: Cambridge University Press.

Kramer, Peter. 1993. *Listening to Prozac.* New York: Penguin.

Lear, Jonathan. 1990. *Love and its Place in Nature: A Philosophical Interpretation of Freudian Psychoanalysis.* New York: Farrar, Straus, and Giroux.

Leichsenring, Falk, and Sven Rabung. 2008. "The Efficacy of Short-Term Psychodynamic Therapy." *Journal of the American Medical Association* 300(13):1551–1565.

Light, Donald. 1980. *Becoming Psychiatrists: The Professional Transformation of Self.* New York: Norton.

———. 2009. "Countervailing Power: The Changing Character of the Medical Profession in the United States." In *The Sociology of Health and Illness*, edited by Peter Conrad, 239–248. New York: Worth.

Light, Donald, and Sol Levine. 1988. "The Changing Character of the Medical Profession: A Theoretical Overview." *Millbank Quarterly* 66(2):10–32.

Luhrmann, T. M. 2001. *Of Two Minds: An Anthropologist Looks at American Psychiatry.* New York: Vintage.

Lunbeck, Elizabeth. 1994. *The Psychiatric Persuasion: Knowledge, Gender, and Power in Modern America*. Princeton, NJ: Princeton University Press.

Marcus, Steven, and Mark Olfson. 2010. "National Trends in the Treatment for Depression 1998–2007." *Archives of General Psychiatry* 67(12):1265–1273.

McGann, P. J., David Hutson, and Barbara Katz Rothman, eds. 2011. *Sociology of Diagnosis: Advances in Medical Sociology* Vol. 12. Bingley, UK: Emerald.

McWilliams, Nancy. 2000. "On Teaching Psychoanalysis in Antianalytic Times: A Polemic." *American Journal of Psychoanalysis* 60:371–390.

———. 2005. "Preserving our Humanity as Therapists." *Psychotherapy: Theory, Research, Practice, Training* 42(2):139–151.

———. 2009. "Some Thoughts on the Survival of Psychoanalytic Practice." *Clinical Social Work Forum* 37:81–83.

Metzl, Jonathan Michel. 2003. *Prozac on the Couch: Prescribing Gender in the Era of Wonder Drugs*. Durham, NC: Duke University Press.

Mishler, Elliot G. 1984. *The Discourse of Medicine: Dialectics of Medical Interviews*. Norwood, NJ: Ablex.

Mojtabai, Ramin, and Mark Olfson. 2008. "National Trends in Psychotherapy by Office-Based Psychiatrists." *Archives of General Psychiatry* 65:962–970.

Moncrieff, Joanna, and Irving Kirsch. 2005. "Efficacy of Antidepressants in Adults." *British Medical Journal* 331:155–157.

Pampallona, Sandro, Paola Bollini, Giuseppe Tibaldi, Bruce Kupelnick, and Carmine Munizza. 2004. "Combined Pharmacotherapy and Psychological Treatment for Depression: A Systematic Review." *Archives of General Psychiatry* 61(7):714–719.

PDM Taskforce. 2006. *Psychodynamic Diagnostic Manual*. Silver Spring, MD: Alliance of Psychoanalytic Organizations.

Porter, Roy. 1997. *The Greatest Benefit to Mankind: A Medical History of Humanity*. New York: Norton.

Pratt, Laura A., Debra J. Brody, and Qiuping Gu. 2011. "NCHS Data Brief: Antidepressant Use in Persons Aged 12 and Over: United States, 2005–2008." National Center for Health Statistics. http://www.cdc.gov/nchs/data/databriefs/db76.htm.

Pratt, Laura A., Debra J. Brody, and Qiuping Gu. 2017. "NCHS Data Brief: Antidepressant Use in Persons Aged 12 and Over: United States, 2011–2014." National Center for Health Statistics. https://files.eric.ed.gov/fulltext/ED575709.pdf.

Rogler, Lloyd H. 1997. "Making Sense of Historical Changes in the Diagnostic and Statistical Manual of Mental Disorders: Five Propositions." *Journal of Health and Social Behavior* 38(1):9–20.

Rose, Nikolas. 2006. "Disorders without Borders: The Expanding Scope of Psychiatric Practice." *BioSocieties* 1:465–484.

Rudnytsky, Peter L. 2000. *Psychoanalytic Conversations: Interviews with Clinicians, Commentators, and Critics*. Hillsdale, NJ: Analytic Press.

Schechter, Kate. 2014. *Illusions of a Future: Psychoanalysis and the Biopolitics of Desire*. Durham, NC: Duke University Press.

Schnittker, Jason. 2017. *The Diagnostic System: Why the Classification of Psychiatric Disorders Is Necessary, Difficult, and Never Settled*. New York: Columbia University Press.

Scull, Andrew. 2015. *Madness in Civilization: A Cultural History of Insanity*. Princeton, NJ: Princeton University Press.

Seligman, Martin E. P. 1995. "The Effectiveness of Psychotherapy: The Consumer Reports Study." *American Psychologist* 50(12):965–974.

Shaw, George Bernard. 1909. *The Doctor's Dilemma: A Tragedy*. New York: Brentano's.

Shorter, Edward. 1993. *From Paralysis to Fatigue: A History of Psychosomatic Illness in the Modern Era.* New York: Free Press.

———. 1997. *A History of Psychiatry: From the Era of the Asylum to the Age of Prozac.* New York: John Wiley.

Smith, Dena T. 2011. A Sociological Alternative to the Psychiatric Conceptualization of Mental Suffering," *Sociology Compass* 5(5):351–363.

Smith, Dena T. 2014. "The Diminished Resistance to Medicalization in Psychiatry: Psychoanalysis Meets the Medical Model of Mental Illness." *Society and Mental Health* 4(2):75–91.

Smith, Dena T., and Jennifer Hemler. 2014. "Classification and Diagnosis." In *Social Issues in Diagnosis: An Introduction for Students and Clinicians,* edited by Annemarie Jutel and Kevin Dew15–32. Baltimore: Johns Hopkins University Press.

Starr, Paul. 1982. *The Social Transformation of American Medicine.* New York: Basic Books.

Strauss, Anselm, Leonard Schatzman, Rue Bucher, Danuta Ehrlich, and Melvin Sabshin. 1981. *Psychiatric Ideologies and Institutions.* New Brunswick, NJ: Transaction.

Timmermans, Stefan, and Marc Berg. 2003a. *The Gold Standard: The Challenge of Evidence-Based Medicine and Standardization in Health Care.* Philadelphia: Temple University Press.

———. 2003b. "The Practice of Medical Technology." *Sociology of Health & Illness* 25(3):97–114.

Whitaker, Robert. 2002. *Mad in America: Bad Science, Bad Medicine, and the Enduring Mistreatment of the Mentally Ill.* Cambridge, MA: Perseus.

Whooley, Owen. 2010. "Diagnostic Ambivalence: Psychiatric Workarounds and the Diagnostic and Statistical Manual of Mental Disorders." *Sociology of Health and Illness* 32:452–469.

Williams, Simon J., Paul Martin, and Jonathan Gabe. 2011. "The Pharmaceuticalization of Society? A Framework for Analysis." *Sociology of Health and Illness* 33(5):710–725.

Zola, Irving Kenneth. 1972. "Medicine as an Institute of Social Control." *American Sociological Review* 20:487–504.

———. 1983. *Socio-medical Inquiries: Recollections. Reflections and Reconsiderations.* Philadelphia: Temple University Press.

Index

Abbott, Andrew, 163

Abilify (antipsychotic), 7

Acute symptoms, medication decision and, 103–107

Allen, Woody, 21

American asylums, 18

American Psychiatric Association: Biodynamic Psychiatrists and, 148; clinical practice guidelines, 30–31; committee on psychotherapy by psychiatrists, 176; DSM and, 23, 29, 76; medications and, 111

American Psychoanalytic Association: Biodynamic Psychiatrists and, 148; on countertransference, 200n3; "Psychoanalytic Lawsuit" and, 33, 198n13; psychoanalytic training institutes and, 32, 33, 200n1; Psychodynamic Psychologists and, 155; on transference, 199n2

Annie Hall (movie), 21

Antidepressants: acknowledgment of limitations of, 178; increasing use of, 6–7, 32; patient response to, 108; practitioners on usefulness of, 110; Prozac, 6–7, 27–28, 170–171; SSRIs, 27–28

Antipsychiatry movement, 16, 198n5, 198n7

Antipsychotic medications, 7, 198n10

Anxiety: DSM-II characterization of, 19–20; DSM-III characterization of, 23; efficacy of psychoanalysis for, 36; psychodynamic therapy for, 116–117

Association of Medical Colleges, 190

Axis I disorders (mood disorders), 32, 85–86, 199n1

Axis II disorders (personality disorders), 32, 85–86, 199n1

Bedside manner, psychoanalytic skills and good, 120–122

Berg, Marc, 9–10, 25–26, 91

Biodynamic Psychiatrists, 139–149: ability to navigate both treatment approaches, 163–164; alignment with one model or another, 161–162; biological and environmental factors in etiology, 99–100; biomedical model and younger cohorts of, 144–145; challenge of expertise and, 140–141; on choice of psychoanalysis for certain patients, 116–117; combined therapy and, 131; on contemporary deficit in psychodynamic training, 119–120; on contribution of psychiatry to society, 117–118; described, 38; different treatments used by, 129–130; difficulty in integrating models, 145–146; on DSM diagnosis, 175; etiology of illness and, 98; freedom and frustration of dual training and, 141–145; identification of, 187; interpersonal tensions with mainstream psychiatrists, 146–149; larger toolkit of, 149; on limitations of psychoanalysis, 124–128; medicalization of psychiatry and, 162; number of patients in practice, 52; on overuse of medications, 108–109, 110, 111, 112–113; portraits of, 39, 49–56; on potential outcomes of medication and psychoanalysis, 118–119; practice composition of, 179; professional identity of, 53–54; psychodynamic psychotherapy and, 113–114, 116–117, 139–140; purpose of medication for, 106–107; questioning biomedical model, 169–170; strategy for medication referrals, 147, 150; training of, 159–161; use of DSM, 64–69, 70–71, 73–75, 78–80, 81, 82–85, 87, 93; on use of medication, 103–104, 106–107; why became psychiatrist, 50–51

Biological vulnerability, as foundation of mental disorder, 3–4

Biology, in etiology of mental illness, 56, 61, 96, 98–99, 100–103

About the Author

Dena T. Smith is an assistant professor of sociology in the Department of Sociology, Anthropology and Health Administration and Policy at University of Maryland, Baltimore County (UMBC). Her research is on the mental health professions and gender and mental health. Her work has appeared in *Society and Mental Health*, *The American Journal of Men's Health*, and *Sociology Compass*.